The Healing Path of Yoga

The Healing Path of Yoga

Time-Honored Wisdom and Scientifically Proven Methods That
ALLEVIATE STRESS, OPEN YOUR HEART, AND
ENRICH YOUR LIFE

NISCHALA JOY DEVI

 THREE RIVERS PRESS • NEW YORK

A NOTE TO THE READER

The information in this book is not intended as a substitute for the advice of physicians or other qualified health professionals. It is not intended to be prescriptive with reference to any specific ailment or condition or to the general health of the reader, but, rather, descriptive of one approach to fostering health and wellness. The reader is advised to consult with his or her physician before undertaking any of the practices contained in this book. The reader should also continue to consult regularly with his or her physician in matters relating to his or her health, particularly in respect to any symptoms that may require diagnosis or medical treatment. Neither the author nor the publisher shall be liable or responsible for any loss, injury, or damage allegedly arising from the use of any information contained in this book.

Published by Three Rivers Press, New York, New York.
Member of the Crown Publishing Group.

Random House, Inc. New York, Toronto, London, Sydney, Auckland
www.randomhouse.com

THREE RIVERS PRESS is a registered trademark and the Three Rivers Press colophon
is a trademark of Random House, Inc.

Printed in the United States of America
Design by Lauren Dong

Library of Congress Cataloging-in-Publication Data

Devi, Nischala Joy.
    The healing path of Yoga : time-honored wisdom and scientifically proven methods
        that alleviate stress, open you heart, and enrich your life / by Nischala Joy
        Devi.—1st ed.
        p.   cm
    1. Yoga, Hatha.   I. Title.
    RA781.7.D485 2000
    613.7'046—dc21

ISBN 0-609-80502-9

10   9   8   7   6   5   4   3   2   1

First Edition

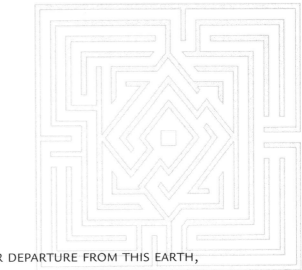

TO MY MOTHER, BELLE,

MY FIRST GURU, WHO, AFTER HER DEPARTURE FROM THIS EARTH,

HAS LEFT ME WITH THE EXPERIENCE AND KNOWLEDGE

THAT UNCONDITIONAL LOVE IS POSSIBLE

ACKNOWLEDGMENTS

THE HEALING PATH OF YOGA is an open-ended journey that began long before I knew there would ever be a book of that name. The courage to even tread on this glorious path was nourished at first by my two remarkable parents, who believed with their whole hearts that I was the greatest blessing in their lives. With their gentle guidance and love they allowed me to be the person I have become. I am sure they are now the ever-present angels guiding me through life.

To my earth angel, the love of my life, best friend, and playmate, Bhaskar Deva, who makes everything in my life more joyous and fun. Even during my tenth rewrite of a chapter his love for me made me smile.

I have been very blessed in my life to have had loving guidance from many people. I know they rejoice with me that this book is now available.

I am forever grateful for the years of insight and guidance into the teachings and practices of yoga that I received from my guru, Sri Swami Satchidananda.

To Dean Ornish, M.D., for believing that a Yoga-based program could reverse heart disease and for taking the time from his extremely busy schedule to write the foreword.

Thanks to Michael Lerner, Ph.D., and the Commonweal Cancer Help Team for the experience and knowledge that I gained in developing and serving that great program.

I learned so much from the members of my clinical team at the Preventive Medicine Research Institute, who patiently listened to my concerns about the physical and subtle bodies not being included in their vast traditional medical training.

All the problem-solving done with yoga teachers, who were teaching people with life-threatening diseases, stocked my mental files, encouraging me to be very creative in my advice.

To my dear friends and cheering section: Gwynn Sullivan; Swamis Vidyananda, Ramananda; Vajra Matasow; Kevin Cates; Lakshmi Fjord, Janet Whitman, and Bill Bilawa, who were among the many people who said, "You should write a book." Especially to Julie Lusk, who not only said it to me, but to her agent, who responded, "I love it, let's publish it!" This was the beginning of my dream team. Combining the skills, love, encouragement, and guidance of my agent, Loretta Barrett, and editor, Shaye Areheart, was like heart and heartbeat. To both of them and their great teams, who skillfully soothed my apprehensions on more than one occasion, for producing a beautiful and inspiring book.

To Kacie Woodard for the preliminary drawings and to Cassi Stish for her grace and skill in excecuting "real people drawings." To Sabina Vogt for the photos and flexibility.

To my dear editor friends, Radihka Miller and Prakash Shakti Capen, whose velvet fingers helped to edit and transform unfinished sentences into readable thoughts.

To my sweet and patient friends Robin Gueth, for her copywriting and publicity tips; Debra Kesten who answered Publishing 101 questions; Jeffrey Kroeber, and Richard Fairbanks for endless help, patience, and mercy for the technically impaired.

To my in-laws, Ronald and Beverly Gross, Dayle, Ken, Emily, and Jordan Myers and Mark Gross, whose love and support of me exemplify the benefits of yoga and change in-law to in-love.

I give a deep and heartfelt bow to all the people with heart disease and other life-threatening diseases who taught me about the healing power of love and compassion. And to those who whispered in my heart, "Tell my story," I thank you for the inspiration.

I bow to those who were courageous enough to try almost anything to help themselves heal. Because of your courage, so much was learned that is now benefiting not just a few but many. I thank you and they thank you.

All who cheered me on and believed in me: If I have not mentioned your name, forgive me, you are always in my heart.

CONTENTS

FOREWORD

FOR THE PAST TWENTY-THREE YEARS, my colleagues and I have conducted a series of cardiovascular studies demonstrating, for the first time, that the progression of even severe coronary heart disease often can be slowed, stopped, or even reversed by a program of comprehensive lifestyle changes, without coronary bypass surgery, angioplasty, or a lifetime of cholesterol-lowering drugs. These lifestyle changes include a very low-fat, whole-food vegetarian diet, stress management techniques, moderate exercise, smoking cessation, and psychosocial support. This was a radical idea when I began my first study; now, it has become mainstream and is generally accepted as true by most cardiologists and scientists.

I have studied yoga since 1972 with Sri Swami Satchidananda, an eminent and ecumenical spiritual teacher and yoga master. Indeed, the "stress management techniques" that are an important part of the program are derived in large part from the yoga and meditation practices that I learned from him.

One of my colleagues has been Nischala Devi. I first began working with her in 1986 at the beginning of the Lifestyle Heart Trial. At that time, she was in charge of teacher training for the Satchidananda Ashram. Along with Sandra McLanahan, M.D., she became one of the primary initial instructors for our research participants and at our weeklong residential retreats.

One of the most important lessons I learned from Swami Satchidananda was to always ask: What is the cause? And what is the cause of that? And so on. The theme of all of our work is simple: If we do not treat the underlying causes of a problem, then the same problem may recur, new problems may emerge, or we may be faced with painful choices. This is like mopping up the floor around an overflowing sink without also turning off the faucet.

Within a few weeks after making comprehensive lifestyle changes, the patients in our research reported a 91-percent average reduction in the frequency of angina. Most of the patients became essentially pain free, including those who had been unable to work or engage in daily activities due to severe chest pain. Within a month, we measured increased blood flow to the heart and improvements in the heart's ability to pump. And within a year, even severely blocked coronary arteries began to improve in 82 percent of the patients.

These research findings were published in the most well-respected peer-reviewed medical journals, including the *Journal of the American Medical Association, The Lancet, Circulation, The New England Journal of Medicine, The American Journal of Cardiology,* and others.

In our latest report, published in the December 16, 1998, issue of the *Journal of the American Medical Association,* we found that most of the study participants were able to maintain comprehensive lifestyle changes for five years. On average, they demonstrated even more reversal of heart disease after five years than after one year. In contrast, the patients in the comparison group who made only the moderate lifestyle changes recommended by most physicians (i.e., a diet with 30 percent of calories coming from fat) worsened after one year, and their coronary arteries became even more clogged after five years. Also, we found that the incidence of cardiac events (e.g., heart attacks, strokes, bypass surgery, and angioplasty) was 2.5 times lower in the group that made comprehensive lifestyle changes after five years.

The next research question was: How practical and cost-effective is this lifestyle program?

There is bipartisan interest in finding ways to control health care costs without compromising the quality of care. Many people are concerned that managed care approaches such as shortening hospital stays, shifting from inpatient to outpatient surgery, and forcing doctors to see more and more patients in less and less time, may compromise the quality of care because they do not address the underlying causes—often lifestyle factors—that often lead to illnesses like coronary heart disease.

Beginning five years ago, my colleagues and I established the Multi-center Lifestyle Demonstration Project. It was designed to determine: (a) if we could train other teams of health professionals in diverse regions of the country to motivate their patients to follow this lifestyle program; (b) if this program may be an equivalently safe and effective alternative to bypass surgery and angioplasty in selected patients with severe but stable coronary artery disease; and (c) the resulting cost savings. In other words, can some patients avoid bypass surgery and angioplasty by making comprehensive lifestyle changes at lower cost without increasing cardiac morbidity and mortality?

In the past, lifestyle changes have been viewed only as *prevention*, increasing costs in the short run for a possible savings years later. Now, this program is offered as a scientifically proven alternative *treatment* to many patients who otherwise were eligible for coronary artery bypass surgery or angioplasty, thereby resulting in an immediate and substantial cost savings.

For every patient who chooses this lifestyle program rather than undergoing bypass surgery or angioplasty, thousands of dollars are immediately saved that otherwise would have been spent; much more when complications occur. (Of course, this does not include sparing the patient the trauma of undergoing cardiac surgery.) Also, providing lifestyle changes as a direct alternative for patients who otherwise would receive coronary bypass surgery or coronary angioplasty may result in significant *long-term* cost savings. Despite the great expense of bypass surgery and angioplasty, up to one-half of bypass grafts reocclude after only five to seven years, and 30 to 50 percent of angioplastied arteries restenose after only four to six months. When this occurs, the coronary bypass surgery or coronary angioplasty is often repeated, thereby incurring additional costs.

Through our nonprofit research institute, the Preventive Medicine Research Institute (PMRI), we trained at a diverse selection of hospitals and other sites around the country. In brief, we found that 77 percent of people who were eligible for bypass surgery or angioplasty were able to avoid it safely by making comprehensive lifestyle changes in the hospitals where we trained. Mutual of Omaha calculated an immediate savings of $29,529 per patient. These patients reported reductions in angina comparable to what can be achieved with bypass surgery or angioplasty, without the costs or risks of surgery. These findings were published in the *American Journal of Cardiology* in November 1998. We also found that patients who needed bypass surgery or angioplasty were able to reduce the likelihood of needing another operation by making comprehensive lifestyle changes after surgery.

The techniques described here by Nischala Devi are much more than strategies to help us cope with, or deal with, or manage, stress. Yoga is a system of dynamic tools for achieving union and healing—with parts of ourselves, with others, and with a higher force. This is a powerful and wise prescription for opening the heart in its deepest sense.

DEAN ORNISH, M.D.
Founder and President, Preventive Medicine Research Institute
Clinical Professor of Medicine
School of Medicine, University of California, San Francisco
author of *Dr. Dean Ornish's Program for Reversing Heart Disease* and *Love & Survival*
www.Ornish.com

The Healing Path of Yoga

Introduction:
How This All Came to Be

STRESS IS NOW CONSIDERED the foremost contributor to our modern chronic maladies. Recent medical research by well-known clinicians has shown that stress is a major factor in causing heart disease, cancer, and a myriad of chronic and acute diseases of today's world.

Physical and mental stress accumulate. This can lead to fatigue, a drop in performance level, and a feeling of anxiety. If not checked, stress creates more serious problems and disease occurs.

Mental and physical dis-ease *or* well-being can be fundamentally improved by acquiring a few simple tension-lowering techniques. Further investigation reports that adherence to yoga-based stress management techniques may be a major determinant in slowing the progression of or reversing these diseases.

This book can show you practical and enjoyable practices and hints that can help transform the *stresses* of daily life into the *joys* of daily life. While the stressful events around us may not change, we can learn how to respond skillfully to life's difficulties, maintaining our equilibrium and a sense of well-being.

Knowing this, I offer my experience—practical and experiential—of

"IT REQUIRES A VERY UNUSUAL MIND TO UNDERTAKE THE ANALYSIS OF THE OBVIOUS."

—*Alfred North Whitehead*

using the ancient art and science of yoga for the total healing of body, mind, and spirit.

Since I grew up with and was originally trained in western medicine yet am very much alive in the spirit, the merging or meshing of the worlds of fact and knowing was less difficult for me than for most. It was a gradual process, yet one incident stands out in my heart and mind.

In 1968, while working as a medical assistant for a cardiologist, I was doing all the peripheral duties that surround a traditional medical practice. The patient would come in and be greeted and asked for any complaints. Problems would be noted on their chart. Routine, weight, blood pressure, EKG, and other tests would be taken.

The patients and I became well acquainted. We would chat, share stories and adventures. One man who was a regular visitor had severe hypertension. When I took his blood pressure on this particular visit, it was dangerously high. I had the idea to have him lie down and relax for a few minutes. While he was relaxing, I asked him to tell me about his summer holidays. What did he enjoy during his time off? He began to tell me in detail about his family being together—going sailing, swimming, and just relaxing. While his eyes were closed in imagination, I noticed he had a smile on his face.

A few minutes later, I took his blood pressure: It had gone way down. Surprise, surprise!

Elated with joy, I rushed into the cardiologist's office and told him the wonderful news. Barely looking up from the chart of another patient, he said, "Raise the medication."

"But," I protested, "his blood pressure came down when he relaxed!"

"So?" said the still-preoccupied doctor.

"Can't we do something else besides raise the medication?"

"Like what?" he asked.

Hopelessly silent, I couldn't find an answer that would offer the man a viable alternative to medication.

The last thirty years has been spent in trying to answer the question: "What else can be done?"

This book is part of that answer.

In 1969, I left traditional medicine and began my own spiritual quest. Looking into many spiritual paths, the complete system of Yoga resonated most within my soul. After much searching, my heart yearned to find a teacher to guide me.

In 1973, my heart led me to the spiritual vibration of Sri Swami Satchidananda. A great and holy Yoga master, his spark ignited and allowed me to renew an ancient commitment. He was to guide me on the inner journey to my soul's song. That journey has also enabled me to merge the knowledge of spirit with ancient healing traditions and modern medicine.

In 1975 and 1977, I accepted an eternal commitment, dedicating my life to the service of humanity by taking vows as a monk in the holy order of Sannyas. In 1991, for personal reasons, I chose to leave the *formal* vows, still keeping the eternal promise to know myself and to serve and love all.

In 1979, while living as a monk, my service drew me to serve at a holistic health center run by the ashram (spiritual community) where I was a member. There I was able to use the practices of yoga in a therapeutic setting. This experience showed me the endless possibilities for strengthening and purifying the body and mind, allowing healing to occur.

In the summer of 1982, I was training yoga students to become teachers. One of the students at the training approached me and told me his dream. He had started a healing center on the California coast and wanted to begin yoga-based retreats for people who had cancer.

How exciting, I thought.

"And," he said, "would you be willing to help develop the yoga part of the program?"

The "yes" could not have come from my tongue any faster. It was a dream come true. The man was Michael Lerner, Ph.D., founder of the Commonweal Cancer Help Program, and that was the beginning of the now famous and award-winning Commonweal Cancer Help Program in Bolinas, California.

Coincidentally, that *same* week another young man, who was a resident physician at the Harvard Medical Center, Massachusetts General Hospital, in Boston, came to the ashram. We had known each other casually, and I knew of the work he was doing while still in medical school with heart patients: He was using yoga practices to help alleviate the pain and symptoms of people suffering from the life-debilitating disease.

Speaking one afternoon on the back lawn, he mentioned that he was about to do a major clinical trial with patients who were rejected from undergoing bypass surgery because of the extent of their disease or other medical complications. One of the major components of the study would be yoga practices. He was looking for someone to help to develop the yoga aspect and teach the patients how to do the practices. Was I interested?

Am I interested? My inner voice rang. It was as if all the service and practices I had done in my life came together in that one week.

Having also committed to doing the Commonweal Cancer Help Program, I realized I needed to make a decision about which I would do.

Why can't you do both? another part of my heart or mind (it was difficult to tell which one) said. After less than a moment, I heard myself saying, "Okay, I'll do both."

The rest is amazing history. The medical resident was Dean Ornish, M.D., president and director of the Preventive Medicine Research Institute, Sausalito, California, and author of the study The Lifestyle Heart Trial, which proved a yoga-based program, along with a lowfat diet, exercise, and group support, could in fact reverse heart disease.

I feel very blessed to have been involved with these two landmark programs.

I worked with The Lifestyle Heart Trial for three years, developing the yoga portion of the program. At the same time my service in other areas was growing. I decided to withdraw temporarily from The Lifestyle Heart Trial and continue my traveling and teaching around the world.

In 1992, I moved back to California and called Dr. Ornish to let him know about my recent move and to ask if there was any service I could do with the continuing study.

The Lifestyle Heart Trial had been so successful that a new study, The Multicenter Lifestyle Heart Trial, was being expanded to include eight hospitals across the United States. Someone was needed to help develop the curriculum, write the manuals, choose and train the yoga teachers. "Are you interested in taking the position of director of stress management?" Dr. Ornish asked. Again my heart chanted, YES!

Now it's time for me to share what I have learned.

Yoga is a complete system of how to live our lives. It leads us to a whole new way of living. It is not a religion, yet it can be combined *with* a religion to increase the richness of any tradition. It was developed as a system

about five thousand years ago. The ancient *Yoga Sutras of Pat*
first book to take the *oral* tradition of Yoga, with its exis
practices, and write it down, allowing the great teachi
accessible, understood, and practiced. Throughout *The I*
I refer to these *Sutras* (literally meaning thread) as a b
the various types of meditation and Yogic technique/

Yoga allows us to bring an expanded conscious
and healing to our everyday activities, starting from tin
bow of practices was developed to help us make that journey. .
that rainbow is the knowledge that *we* are the healers. Taking respo.
bility for our own health and well-being, our bodies and minds reveal the
secrets of balance, harmony, and the release of energy for healing. This
decreases the need for someone else to "fix us." We learn more about our
bodies and minds than anyone else. We then consult with professionals as
partners in our healing process, not as fixers.

Even some modern medical practices come from ancient Yogic techniques. On a recent visit to a doctor about her back pain, my friend
reported she was given "yogalike" exercises. Many of the natural child-
birth techniques borrow the deep relaxation technique of tightening one
muscle group while the rest of the body remains relaxed. In hospitals
postoperative patients are routinely taught how to breathe deeply using
the belly. Yoga allows us to be our own healers.

Over the years I have worked with hundreds and hundreds of people
with various degrees of problems and illnesses. Some came because they
were suffering from the common modern-day catchall, stress. They asked
for "just one technique that would work to cure me," something simple
to do that would take away their back pain, headaches, and even cancer.
We are not simple beings. In fact, we are very complex. A simple back pain
is not so simple. It is composed of how we use or abuse the muscles, how
we think, feel, eat, sleep, and rest. Are we able to acknowledge and even
touch the essence of who we are?

To use the ancient techniques of Yoga is to use them as a complete system. As Yoga became popular in this country some forty years ago, it was
dissected. The *physical poses* were embraced by those who were more physically oriented and who liked to move and stretch the body. *Breathing practices* were studied by those needing to increase their oxygen capacity.

Meditation techniques were developed as a means for deepening the intellect and inner strength. The *vegetarian diet* was adapted by the back-to-the-earth folks and pacifists.

It concerns me when I read, see, or hear a "natural and holistic" health practitioner who dissects the ancient practices and prescribes them as if they were drugs. "Take three minutes of shoulder stand, two neck movements, three deep breaths, and a glass of pure filtered water and call me in a week. This should make you all better." When we do this and do not get better, we feel that natural methods do not work. How long did it take you to get sick? How many years of stress and emotional buildup? All that *cannot* be changed overnight. Even in the case of complete cures, if the right lifestyle is not followed the disease is likely to return. Yoga is not a *treatment,* it is a *consciousness* that allows health, balance, and joy to be your companions throughout your entire life's journey.

Now is the time to recognize the ancient system as a whole, a new, old way to live, a lifestyle change that can allow you to feel that joy for living. It can make a difference in your personal life *and* in the greater world community.

Use and experience this book and its recommended consciousness and lifestyle changes as a whole. The seemingly unusual ideas and practices will become more comfortable as you are able to see them in totality with your life. The purpose of the book is to make you *more comfortable with yourself.* This is the same advice I offer to my students and clients, the same advice I incorporate into my own life.

If you are more scientifically minded, you may ask, "Where is the proof?" The results you experience are the proof and they are usually dramatic. Many heart and cancer patients would quietly and secretly confess to me that it was the yoga as stress management portion of the program they needed the most. Then over time they would echo, "How could something so simple make such a dramatic change?" Many times the practice that seems the most difficult is the one we need the most. Instead of trusting someone else's research findings, make your own body and mind the laboratory. Amaze yourself at the results.

Many of us think of our lives as a mathematical equation: They start at point A and go in a straight line to point B. We are born at point A and we die at point B. In between are just a series of dots or events. We go to school, marry, have children, retire, and before we know it we are at point

B. If we fail to travel in that straight line we think of ourselves as having failed. "If I do not have children by the time I am thirty-five, what will become of me? It will be too late." "After all these years I am still working in the same department! What is wrong with me?" Life is not a straight line; it is a circular journey that has the journey itself as the goal. Stopping to enjoy a sunset, being present for our child's first word, the smell of bread coming out of the oven are some of the *small* accomplishments and treasures that make our lives rich and personal. Sometimes we may choose to take the scenic route, sometimes we stay with the perceived straight way. We may not be able to change outside circumstances, yet we can choose not to feel victimized by the direction that our lives take. Instead, we can see each step as an exciting new adventure.

A retired fighter pilot was feeling remorse about the circuitous course his healing process was taking. My husband, Bhaskar Deva, a fellow pilot, was giving some advice, using the analogy of navigational techniques to make his point. "If you want to go from San Francisco to New York, we plot a straight line on the map," said Bhaskar. "It is not possible for an airplane to fly from point A to point B without compensating for cross-winds. Even when our goal is to the east, we must adjust the heading and fly north or south, seemingly away from the goal. It may look as if we are off course or even going the wrong way when we are actually right on track. The constant corrections are the most effective way to reach our goal. It is nice to enjoy all the sights along the way *and* the journey. So, according to this way of thinking, you really *have been* on course all these years."

Regardless of our age or the condition of our health, there comes a time in our lives when we draw away from the outward and move inward. This book is about the journey to find our true self, the path of our heart, through life's labyrinth.

A labyrinth is a series of paths and passages that wind in and out of life's adventures without a direct route. We find our own way into our own center and from there back out again. Learning as we go, these passages represent the different aspects of our lives. To some, life seems to change quickly; to others, more slowly. Many people who are coping with life-threatening illnesses tend to quicken their inward movement. The practices of Yoga can help gently guide us toward the learning and awareness life has to teach us. Sometimes they can help us find new perceptions and understand life's lessons more quickly. We may be able to avoid the prolongation of pain and suffering.

Many great transformations I have experienced in people have come through attitude changes. Sometimes, the tougher people seem and the more they resist looking into themselves, the deeper inward they are eventually able to go.

One such man stays in my heart from one of the earlier Reversing Heart Disease residential retreats. On the first day when we shared how each person came to the program, this man grumpily answered, "My wife made me come." Well, anyone in the room could see this was not the kind of man who sheepishly did whatever his wife wished. On further admission, he was losing his ability to lead what he considered a normal, active life. His heart, weakened by two heart attacks and three bypass operations, was no longer able to supply the body with its needed quantity of blood. This retreat had become the court of last resort.

Each morning as he would enter the yoga classroom he would greet me by flashing the two-fingered peace sign that was so popular in the 1960s and the words "*Peace,* sister." The sarcastic vibration far outweighed the vibration of peace.

This same greeting lasted for a few days. On the afternoon of the third day after the deep relaxation I noticed that this man did not sit up when the rest of the group did. I quietly went over to him to make sure he was all right. It was not so uncommon for a deep sleep to occur and continue throughout and even to the end of class.

He opened his eyelids halfway. "Are you okay?" I asked. A slight fluttering of his upper lids put my mind at ease. I stayed near him as I conducted the final portion of the class. By this time his lids were in the open position and his energy was back in his physical body.

I waited in silence so as not to change the focus of this moment. "I don't know what happened," he began. "I was still me but somehow I was . . . I don't even know how to describe it . . . well, everything seemed right."

Not wanting to put words in his mouth, I said quietly, "Peaceful."

"Yeah, maybe it was peaceful," he replied.

After some time he slowly left the room. When I saw him the next morning, I expected his usual greeting. The gesture was the same, but the tone was completely different. The *peace* was emphasized and the *sister* was sweetened. His view was changed.

In the space and aeronautics field as a spaceship goes up it gains *altitude*. If you look out of the window you may not see the moon. If the ship rotates it is called changing *attitude*. With an attitude change you can now see the moon.

The attitude of this man was changed by his new view of himself and the world. His view also helped to influence a large insurance company to make the Dr. Dean Ornish Reversing Heart Disease program a defined benefit, which then paved the way for other insurance companies to follow. Change the attitude of one and the whole world can change.

Beginning the journey through the labyrinth, starting at the outer edge, we slowly wind back and forth, moving inward to a quiet and still place—the very center of our being. Pausing for a time, we meander back to the outer edges with a greater understanding of ourselves and the world. We then go back in for yet a deeper insight. The process is continuous and without goal. Yet, each time we touch our very center, we are changed.

Acting as a labyrinth, this book begins at the outer edge with Chapter 1, Heart to Heart. In this familiar aspect of our lives, we learn to cherish ourselves as we interact with others at home, work, and play even as we do the necessary chores of daily life. How we feel and act toward others and how they project their feelings toward us becomes our touchstone. The awareness of observing how our actions, words, and thoughts affect us and others is a gift. We are able to observe who we are in the world and assess our strengths and weaknesses. Are we the person we want to be? Kind and loving? Strong and powerful? Perhaps both at the same time?

Moving inward in Chapter 2, Thinking Makes It So—Imagery. Through the practice of imagery we begin to unravel how our actions and thoughts mold our lives. We assess our lives and observe how our inner actions affect our health and happiness. Through our conscious images we are able to manifest the quality of life we desire. Imagery becomes a familiar tool that can transform a difficult or painful situation into a time of growth and understanding. Imagery can transform our *entire* life.

We move further inward in Chapter 3, Deep Rest, Deep Relaxation. So much of our energy goes outward it is necessary to recharge and totally relax, a real deep relaxation. We discover the web of energy that surrounds us and is within us. The quiet knowledge within emerges, encouraging us to take a portion of our day to relax deeply and let go of tension.

Relaxation breaks replace coffee breaks. The body and mind are revitalized. Life seems more easeful.

As the body relaxes, we are able to move further inward in Chapter 4,
The Affirmation of Life—Breath. We tap into the vast wellspring of vital
energy within the breath and experience it as more than just the air we
breathe. It becomes the affirmation of our very life, that which connects
us to the earth and to every living thing on the earth. We open to the
knowledge of this life energy and harness it for the purposes of healing,
enhancing our relationships, directing our careers and our overall well-
being.

Following the life force, we find ourselves in the center of the
labyrinth and seeking to know our true self. At the center, in Chapter 5,
Dynamic Stillness—Meditation, we learn, practice, and experience meditation. It seems that all the steps that led us to the center were necessary
to achieve the quiet and stillness of body and mind. Touching our center
even for an instant, nothing is ever quite the same again. Our life's course
has been corrected and with that realization the journey takes us outward
again.

In Chapter 6, Move and Heal—Physical Poses, we experience the physical body as a complex instrument governed by many things. It no longer
is thought of as a bag of bones, muscles, or a nuisance that causes us pain
or slows us down. If treated with respect, the energy flows through the
body without impediment. We let go of the strain and stress acquired in
the name of efficiency and productivity. By gently positioning the body in
various poses, we allow it to realign with its own natural energy, weaving
an awareness of comfort uniting body, mind, and spirit. The result is
healing and wholeness. A body of health and strength becomes a reality.

On our outward journey we are given instructions on the care and
feeding of the body and mind in Chapter 7, Eating for Wholeness. This
information was given to us on our arrival on this earth, yet like many
instruction booklets, many of us chose not to read it. This time we take
the time to ask our bodies and minds what food and fuel is most beneficial. We are highly refined beings and for best efficiency only the highest
quality food can be used. We become conscious of the multidimensional
nourishment food can give us. Our eating habits come into balance . . .
our bodies and minds become fit for life.

The fitness is manifested in our ability to sleep deeply in Chapter 8,

Prelude to Sleep. Sleeping in the still of the night, our bodies and minds carry on a deep cleansing process. What a joy to be able to rise up in the morning with the vitality of a child and move outward to an exciting and promising day! This is something many of us wish for, a wish that can be granted and realized quickly through simple practices.

We once more find ourselves at the outward rim of the labyrinth at a different place from where we started, again viewing ourselves and our lives. From here we are able to assess the benefit of a yogic lifestyle, yet may doubt our success in accomplishing the changes. We come up with excuses, doubts, and fears. In Chapter 9, Great Excuses, Great Solutions, we will learn how to adjust our already busy day to include a time for practice as well as simple suggestions that can transform our lives into an enjoyable adventure.

I wish you a great and peaceful journey.

"[EVERYONE] SHOULD STRIVE TO LEARN BEFORE THEY DIE WHAT THEY ARE RUNNING FROM, AND TO, AND WHY."

—*James Thurber*

CHAPTER 1

Heart to Heart

A SINGLE HEART CELL was taken from the heart of one person. It continued to beat as an individual cell representing the whole heart. It made the sound *bliiip blop*. Another single cell was taken from a different person's heart. It made the sound *blip blooop*.

In a laboratory-controlled situation, each of these cells was placed in a petri dish. They continued to beat as before: *Bliiip blop, blip blooop*. The dishes were moved close together. Then one of the cells was carefully transferred to the other's dish. At the very instant the two cells—foreigners to each other—touched, they ceased to beat. At the very next instant, they started to beat in unison to a totally different rhythm: *Bliiip blooop, bliiip blooop*. The two cells now danced to the same rhythm. Our individual heart cells, like the members of a well-tuned orchestra, beat as one.

We are part of the whole body of humanity, living in our own worlds, surrounded by life's dreams and dramas. To touch and embrace another allows us to feel the rhythm of our *own* heart.

An abstract artist from a communist country in Eastern Europe and a practical Afro-American preschool teacher from a large, urban city were about to have their hearts heal and beat as one. He was prejudiced against

> "IN NOTHING DO [HUMANS] MORE NEARLY APPROACH THE GODS THAN IN DOING GOOD TO THEIR FELLOW [BEINGS]."
>
> —*Cicero*

anyone who was not white. She wanted to make friends and soothe any-one she could. All week he avoided her glances and smiles, sitting as far from her as the small, intimate room would allow. Their common enemy was cancer.

He had narrowly escaped the invasion of his country by swimming to safety. Could he now escape the invasion of his body by the foreign cells?

Her genes held the memory of oppression, slavery, and injustice. These two people actually had more in common than cancer.

As fate would have it, every person was paired up for the healing touch exercise, leaving the two of them odd couple out. He seemed to have visu-ally withdrawn into his body with a shudder and stiffening. She opened with delight; her chance to get close to him now appeared.

The person lying down received the healing energy while the other person sitting beside them was the transmitter. Unable to contain his dis-dain, he laid down first. With an open heart, she first placed her hands together in a prayer position and then, asking her partner's permission, placed them on his diseased pancreas.

The magic could be felt in the entire room. Love and compassion seemed to permeate every cell and thought. The healing energy leapt across continents and racial barriers, religions and prejudices. The spon-taneity of hearts healing melted the frozen hatred. As they embraced, tears flowed from both sets of eyes. We all formed a circle around their new-found openness. A healing greater than *themselves* had taken place.

The human heart functions on many levels. The best known is its dra-matic and selfless work as a pump and supplier of blood to the entire body. Science is now realizing what the mystics and poets have known for eternity: that the heart is more than a mechanical pump.

One of the latest risk factors for heart disease, cancer, and other chronic life-threatening diseases is the apparent isolation we, as a western culture, find ourselves experiencing on a daily basis.

For the interest of career, education, climate change, or just new hori-zons, we remove ourselves from the familiar. When the move occurs, shift-ing our support system, our hearts tend, at least temporarily, to toughen. The comfort of home, family, and friends is traded for excitement and challenge.

These unfamiliar circumstances make it increasingly painful to keep an open heart. Living in the same place for a whole lifetime was the norm until recently. The suffering we experienced was usually doled out in small amounts over a period of time. Our heartaches were limited by the number of people we knew. When we learned that a man across town had a terrible accident, we may have felt a fleeting sadness. Taking a moment to be thankful that it was not one of our family or close friends, we then went on with the rest of our day.

We have a great capacity to adapt to even the worst of circumstances and, after a while, that heartache fades into the background. The heart, a little less open, may go unnoticed.

In ancient times, we were only able to travel as far as we could by walking. Then, as animals were trained to carry us, our world expanded. With the advent of the automobile, airplane, and now spaceship, our boundaries seem limitless.

Talking with someone across the world is as simple as if they are next door. Many of us do not even *know* the people next door—their sorrows and joys, hopes and dreams. With the addition of the computer age, it becomes safer for us to share intimate details with strangers we will never meet and whose real names we don't even know than our next-door neighbors.

Do you remember the first time you went away from home? You might have been stricken with the disease called homesickness. This disease tends to lessen with each subsequent trip away. When moving to a new "home" it takes some time till it becomes rich with friends and comfort. After a while the familiarity the "new" home allows makes the "old" home easier to leave. Still, the most traveled holiday in the United States today is Thanksgiving—a family holiday—a time to go *home*.

The horrific events on TV seem to harden us, close our hearts. The evening news and magazine programs take us like voyeurs into private and intimate moments of death, destruction, and even birth all over the world. We see and hear details that only one's closest family members would have known about before these modern times. We try to detach and protect ourselves from the knowledge that we are all one family, that *their* pain is *our* pain. To avoid feeling the pain, our emotional hearts contract like the iris of the eye. It is interesting that we are not able to accommodate the overwhelming pain and sadness in our hearts when a large number of people are being hurt or killed. Knowing this, the news media, when reporting a catastrophic event, may choose to focus on one or two individuals. As our hearts feel compassion for those individuals, we are able to slowly expand our empathy and embrace the sufferings of the larger body of humanity.

Talking with my travel agent on the phone one afternoon, I was suddenly stricken with a strange sensation in my body. I could not pinpoint a pain, just a general feeling of "all is not well." Hanging up the phone, I went to lie down. I fell into a deep sleep and awoke to feel very drained of energy. I managed to get to the kitchen for some water. The TV was on and there was a special announcement: An airliner carrying more than two hundred people on board had crashed. There were no survivors. On investigation I found that it had happened about the same time I had felt the "drain of energy." Coincidence? Maybe. Maybe not.

Could we all be connected by the same thread of life energy? When a disaster happens and many die, is the whole force field shaken?

Our trust and faith in each other dwindles with our expanded lives. Pledging our love and getting married now takes on the look of a business merger: "I love you now. If in three years we should get divorced, I want this money back that I made. First, sign this paper, then say 'I do.' "

When the community stays small and trust is the contract, life can be more simply conducted.

In certain European countries, the diamond industry is controlled by a small group of Orthodox Jews. In our complicated world of contracts, forms, and security, it is amazing to see that they still keep business transactions simple, because they are based on trust and good faith. They exchange and sell thousands of dollars of diamonds (which they carry in their coat pockets) with a simple handshake and the Hebrew words *Mazel Tov* (Good Luck).

Nothing is ever written down; it is a person's word that is the bond. What happens if a bad deal is made or the incorrect diamond has been sold or even if it is found to be a fake? How would the innocent victim be avenged? Could that be proven? If there are any discrepancies or anyone should try to cheat another, they may be brought in front of their own council of rabbis. If found guilty, they can be given a severe punishment: to be totally ostracized from their friends, extended family, and community. They and their immediate families are deprived of the most important aspect of life, love. Just the threat of that is enough to keep everyone honest.

In our greater society we are faced with a similar type of punishment.

When in prison, a person may only be kept in solitary confinement for a certain prescribed time. Prolonging this period is considered cruel and unusual punishment. It is interesting that being left alone with our own mind is considered an "unusual" punishment. Many a monk would consider it a dream come true. For most criminals it becomes their worst nightmare. Calm minds crave it; tumultuous minds fear it.

We All Like to Be Stroked

Rabbits were being tested to see how their bodies responded to being fed large quantities of foods high in cholesterol. (Rabbits are, by nature, vegetarians.) They were kept in cages (isolation) and fed this food once a day. At the end of the study, it was observed that the rabbits on the top level had higher cholesterol levels than the ones on the bottom level.

The concerned researchers made a thorough investigation as to proper preparation and amount of food given to the rabbits. The mystery remained unsolved. Observing the rabbits being fed, the researchers noticed that the caring young (and very short) assistant had to stand on tiptoes to feed the rabbits on the top-level cages. As she repeated the feeding ritual with the bottom-level cages, she was easily able to reach into the cages. Along with the physical food, she would take the rabbits out of the cage and pet them while murmuring sweet nothings to them. This petting time had become as much a part of the routine as the food. It was difficult to believe that by daily communion with the lab assistant the cholesterol levels in the rabbits were decreased. Yet this was the only thing that was different between the two rows of cages. Stroking a pet is known to lower our blood pressure. It has even been noted to decrease blood pressure in a person whose pet is not a live one but a cute cuddly stuffed animal! We all receive benefit from loving and being loved and stroking and being stroked.

There have been several other studies with premature babies in incubators. It's a difficult way to spend the first days in this world—in a plastic box. When the babies were held and stroked, they gained weight faster, had fewer complications, and could leave the "box" sooner. Failure to thrive is a real disease in which our bodies do not grow or heal, not because of any apparent organic reason, but for lack of emotional support—not just for little babies, but even big grown-up babies.

There Is More to Yoga Than Stretches

Occasionally, I see or hear about heart patients who are following a yoga, stress management, and dietary regime and the results are not good. Their cholesterol, blood pressure, or chest pain is still above normal.

Why is this not working for them? It is not just a matter of *doing* a yoga program or of going through the motions. The poses, breathing, and meditation are practices that draw us inward. They must be balanced with the external. How do we treat or mistreat our own bodies and minds? How do we treat others? How do we live our lives? Are we listening to our hearts or closing out the messages they are giving us?

Judgment of others can lead us to close our hearts. Even if someone is a criminal, convicted of murder, we may condemn what he or she did and give a suitable punishment. However, if we withhold our love and close our heart, we are punishing ourselves as well as them.

As a young prince, Siddhartha was kept within the palace walls, protected from seeing the normal, everyday suffering of humanity. When he ventured out, his heart was torn apart by what had been hidden from him. Leaving his safe refuge, he set out to find the "truth." As the Enlightened One, Buddha, he proclaimed that all life is suffering. This was not a statement of fact but rather an observation. He realized and taught others that the only place to take refuge is deep within our own selves.

The path to this refuge is to love and be loved. Serve others and learn to open to being served.

I, Me, Mine

As young babies we have an open, loving view of the world. When we are fed, warm, and dry, we are happy. We give and accept love readily. Our hearts are wide open. That is one of the reasons most of us enjoy being around young babies.

Somewhere around the age of two, as we begin to identify with our exterior selves and environment, we become more ego centered. At the same time our developing language skills reflect our inner state. "No! No, I won't do that." We begin to identify everything as "mine."

Our parents try to tell us to share and give. Sometimes their actions are a stronger lesson than what they say. For the rest of our lives we are more or less entrenched in the "I, me, mine" thinking. On the few occasions when we say "you" or even "thou," we may notice that we feel happier, more content. As long as we continue to possess and then anticipate the fear of loss, our hearts are contracted.

The Hungarian language, I am told, does not have a general word for "I." The sentence structure implies by the verb ending who is being referred to. If children use the royal *I,* they are scolded and told they are egotistical. Those who learn to speak English or French find that the more they speak a western language, the more self-centered they become. It seems to have something to do with the use of the pronoun *I.* I have tried to speak and write in English without an *I* or *me.* It is very difficult to communicate and be understood. Is being ego centered inherent in western languages?

In a study done in the mid 1970s to 1980s, Larry Schwerwitz, Ph.D., now director of research at the Complementary Medicine Research Institute, California Pacific Medical Center, and colleagues discovered an aspect of Type A behavior that appeared to raise individuals' risk for heart disease. They found that Type A students who referred to themselves more frequently using the words *I, me, my,* and *mine* had a much higher blood pressure response than Type A's who referred to themselves less frequently.

As Sri Swami Satchidananda so eloquently says, "If you surround yourself with lots of mines, be careful; they may explode."

The Hand in Service

All the great religions and spiritual systems of the world tell us that when we offer service to those less fortunate, we purify our hearts. When our hearts are pure, we know who we really are. The Bible says, "Blessed are the pure in heart, for they shall know God."

In the West, yoga is best known as Hatha Yoga (the physical aspect). Karma Yoga (service) and Bhakti Yoga (devotion) are the most commonly practiced forms of yoga in other parts of the world. When all are practiced together, they form the team of head, hand, and heart.

Karma means "action," the law of action and reaction: "As you sow, so you shall reap." Another example from the Bible, "An eye for an eye, a tooth for a tooth," seems also to explain karma. But as Martin Luther King, Jr., so eloquently put it, ". . . if we keep that up we will all be blind and toothless."

Whether we believe in it or not, we all are bound up in karma. Sometimes we see the results directly, sometimes indirectly or not at all. Many of us like to take credit for the "good" karma and blame the "bad" karma on others or on "luck." Sometimes we attribute good and bad luck to a higher power.

If that deal came through with ease, *I did my homework and put a great proposal together.* The more expanded of us may think, *This was my lucky day. God is shining down on me.* If we "lost" the chance of getting a promotion we may revert back to the ego position of "poor me": *The boss likes her better than me, even though I am better suited for the position* or *I have rotten luck. Nothing good ever happens to me.*

The way to be free of the cycles of action and reaction is to put others' feelings and actions in front of our own.

When we compete against others or say unkind words, we are the ones that must look into the sad faces, feel their sense of loss. We may feel great after our victory, yet part of our heart constricts at another's misfortune.

Karma Yoga tempers the law of karma (action and reaction) by redirecting the cycle through selfless service to humanity. If we must reap what we sow, let us sow seeds of a sweet and tasty fruit.

There are as many ways to serve as there are people to serve and be served. Traditional Karma Yoga is doing the best we can and neither expecting nor waiting for praise or blame, much like the old TV show, *The Lone Ranger.* After doing a heroic action, the Lone Ranger would ride off into the sunset, leaving people to say, "We didn't even thank him for what he did. Who was that masked man?" Learning to do the deed for the sake of doing, not for the reward, we may, as a side effect, feel gratified in seeing others happy.

Before we can begin to give selflessly, our hearts must begin to open, to recognize another person's needs. We then honor them by listening to what they need and providing that rather than our opinion of what they *should* do. As our hearts open further, we are able to aid them without judgment and bathe them in compassion, allowing their dignity to be preserved. This kind of giving benefits both giver and receiver.

"Feed a man a fish and he eats for one day. Teach a man to fish and he eats for a lifetime." A familiar saying, yet in order for someone to be taught anything, we must first make sure he has enough to eat at this very moment. "It is difficult to teach a starving man how to fish. Feed them first and then teach them," said Jesus.

As a small child, I was fortunate to be raised in a middle-class family. We were not wealthy, yet we always had enough. It was a family tradition to go to a fancy restaurant in the center of the city on Christmas Day. I loved getting all dressed up in my best clothes, feeling plush carpet and cushy chairs and eating the soft steamy rolls. I felt *very* special on that day.

My father was very gracious and generous, and nothing was spared on this occasion. What was even more special was the one enroute stop we made.

He would purposely drive through the nonposh portion of town. As we neared our first destination, my father would slow the car down to 5 mph. "Look," he would point, "see all of those people waiting in line in the cold?"

"Yes, Daddy."

"They are not as fortunate as we are. They must stand in line waiting for a simple bowl of soup. Always remember there are people who are less fortunate than you. Be thankful for what you have and serve others whenever you can."

It was probably these Christmas "outings" that led me, many years later, to spend my holidays serving food in homeless shelters to people less fortunate.

Some of my greatest holiday memories were in giving to others.

The Gift of Giving

In many countries and traditions the first part of any harvest or even the first part of the weekly earnings are given to the church, temple, or charity. In this way, we are offering the fruits of our labor to the greater good.

It is a way of life to remember others first. To offer the fruits of our own harvest for the benefit of all is the *essence* of Karma Yoga. Even if the offering is done in the mind or heart as a prayer of gratitude—that is aligning with the *spirit* of Karma Yoga.

Did you ever have a fruit tree that produced a great crop? Didn't you want to give some of the fruits to all your friends? Giving to others feels really good. We just need to stretch that concept, even when we might not have an abundance. If we give even when we feel we may not have enough, it is likely that we experience abundance in return. The reward may come as a feeling of satisfaction at having expanded beyond our boundaries, our comfort zone. It becomes an offering of thankfulness to unseen forces.

To begin the path of service, there are many great reputable organizations that we can participate in and support by giving money and/or time anonymously. It is not necessary to do hands-on service right away if that is not your temperament. Raising money for a good cause enables us to begin serving others in a comfortable way.

When our ashram first moved to rural Virginia, we were city people transplanted to the country. The folks around us were simple, and some of them were very poor. For the first couple of years, we were so focused on our survival that all we could think of was, "I, me, mine" or, in this case, "We, us, ours."

After several Christmases of gift giving, we realized that while the "spirit" was appreciated, many of the gifts were not needed or used. Many of the discarded presents were ultimately given to charity collections some weeks later. Each year we vowed not to give gifts the next year. This vow was usually forgotten by the next November.

One year as November came around, our teacher, Sri Swami Satchidananda met with us to "discuss" Christmas. Abundance had been with each of us that year and we did not really need anything more. Embracing the real spirit of Christmas, we reached out into the greater community. And what fun it was.

Each of us took the money we would have spent on giving gifts to each other and put it in a large fund. From that fund a certain amount was used to buy special holiday foods, cheeses, cookies, and festive treats that many of the local families were unable to afford. Always there were toys for the children and special gifts for the mothers and fathers.

Our group would meet for a wrapping party with Christmas carols and good cheer. Then the real fun would begin. We would dress up like Santa and his elves. I am proud to say I was almost a genuine elf with big red cheeks, a red outfit, and a smile from ear to ear.

Santa and his elves are usually depicted traveling by sleigh, but in Buckingham County they traveled by van. I can still see the faces of the children when Santa and company drove up to the small shacks and shanties. I don't know who was more delighted, us or them. Giving can open the heart faster than Santa traveling on Christmas eve.

The next step in giving might be to begin to give more of yourself on an individual basis. You may not be the Mother Teresa type, yet you can find ways and people to serve. I have known of very successful business-people who go and share their skills with some young hopefuls in a poverty-stricken area. The Peace Corps helps us share our skills in countries where there is less technological development. When we share we are also able to learn about the qualities of others. We feel enriched and it sets the tone for the rest of our life.

A client of mine was complaining that even though he was doing everything "right," his heart disease and diabetes were not getting any better. After our meeting, I confirmed that he was indeed "doing it right." It was another skill that this very successful man had mastered. He spoke about his life. He had it very controlled and it was centered on business first; he and his family tied for second place. There was no room for anyone else.

He was desperate to feel better. I asked him if he did any service and he proudly told me that he was patron to many charities. "Do you ever really give of yourself?" I gingerly asked.

"I give of myself through my money," he answered.

"Let's try an experiment," I suggested. "For the next month, at least once a week, go to a local hospital and spend one to two hours in the children's ward." He looked a bit surprised. From experience, I knew the fastest way to open a heart is through a sick child's eyes.

Within two weeks he called and said it was miraculous. His insulin requirements had dropped along with the frequency of his chest pain. The depression that he'd had for months was lifting. "The children, the children. Their faces are so sweet, so loving. I want to go there every day. It makes me feel so good."

When our heart can touch another, two hearts beat as one.

The Heart and Love

As we begin to truly understand the essence of Karma Yoga and service, we realize that doing it without love is like trying to bake bread without grain.

Bhakti Yoga, the yoga of love and devotion, is often thought to be only for the highly emotional temperament. It conjures up images of someone crying or chanting in rapture in front of an altar or image of the Divine. That *can* be an aspect of devotion. But don't confuse *devotion* with *emotion*. True devotion and love are not only shown to the unseen divine but to the divine in every being as well.

Through the onset of disease and the miracle of healing, we begin to rely on the cosmic energy. Twelve Step programs help ease us out of addictive behaviors, asking as the first step to invite a higher power into our lives to help us. We all need help from the higher power above and from each other right here on earth.

Most of us begin our path of devotion by acknowledging there is something beyond the small "i." If we pray for a sick friend or bless them when they sneeze, can we then extend and send blessings to a larger circle of people? The effects of long-distance healing is now becoming commonly known. Even if we do not do it formally, it is always nice to send out our good wishes.

Blessing by touch is one of the oldest healing techniques known. It is believed by ancient healing arts that the energy flows from the heart down the arms and into the hands. Any parent knows the power of touch when consoling a small child. The simple act of placing your hand on a person's arm can bring a message of calmness, sympathy, or caring. An embrace can express something stronger than many words. It can be an expression of "I am sorry," "I am happy to see you," even "I love you."

A touch is not only something we do with the hands; a touch with the eyes can relay healing and love as can a soft word, a smile, or even a thought.

Overnight Train to Moscow

There is a wonderful Russian saying: "To think with the heart is to feel with the mind." Keep the superhighway flowing in both directions.

Our group was at a conference center in northern Finland for a briefing on what to expect traveling into what was, at that time, communist Russia. We were a group of healers and clergy from across the United States about to venture into still-forbidden territory to meet our counterparts who worked for the good of Mother Russia. The excitement and expectation were peaking. Tomorrow we would go back to Helsinki and take an overnight train into Russia and on to Moscow. We had been sharing hopes and fears of what we had heard and what it could be like. Some of the families left at home were fearful of loved ones going into the unknown.

Each country has its restrictions as to what is permitted to pass through the borders. Some countries mainly look for drugs, others firearms and explosives. For Russia, religious and political articles were forbidden. We were all asked to bring gifts for distribution and were told specifically not to bring anything that might be *construed as religious or political propaganda.*

One kind man had used his own money to print up 1500 buttons, some with the word MIR (peace) and others with I LOVE YOU in both English and Russian. He asked each of us, in case it could be misconstrued as political or spiritual goods, to take a quantity and place them in each of our suitcases and carry-ons.

I was not in any way interested in carrying the buttons that I perceived as silly. I certainly had no intention of wearing one. I was much too dignified and sophisticated to do that.

As life would have it, the "button man" was my next-door neighbor at the hotel. I tried to sneak by him when I went to breakfast the day of departure, but he appeared at his door with plastic bags filled with buttons. "Please help carry these beyond the borders," he pleaded. My heart opened where my head balked. I reluctantly took the bag, went back to my room, and stashed it in the very bottom of my carry-on.

It was time to go on our adventure and I slung my knapsack over my shoulder, the contraband buttons only a memory. I was on my way.

It was black as coal when our train ground to a stop at the Finnish-Russian border. The Finnish engine needed to be swapped for a Russian engine so that we could continue our journey. The train would be boarded by Russian soldiers, our passports and visas would be scrutinized, and our bags carefully inspected.

I peered out the window for a glimpse at the people I had been taught to fear since childhood, hiding under our desks at school because the Russians might come and bomb our town. Who are these people that are so evil they would scare little innocent children? I was now getting my first look.

They did look ominous in their uniforms, with their machine guns and big German shepherd dogs. I noticed my heart beating faster and my palms sweating as the footsteps got closer.

The door to my cabin opened, and the enemy and I were face to face. Except he did not look like an enemy, he looked like a sweet young man with deep blue eyes. I remembered that saying from the Revolutionary War "Don't shoot till you see the whites of their eyes." I now knew why the saying was so notable. When you get that close and look into someone's eyes, it may be more difficult to see him as an enemy. He then becomes a person with thoughts, hopes, and fears—just like you.

The soldier came in and, after examining my passport and visa, started going through my luggage. I was still a bit flustered by the looks of the "enemy," and I paid little attention to what he was doing. Then I remembered the buttons. What would happen when he found them? They were not my idea to start with. I was silently working myself up into quite an unpleasant state.

Meanwhile, he was rummaging through the sack his head was halfway in. Then I heard three little words that made my heart explode with joy and changed my entire life. "I love you," he said.

I couldn't believe what I was hearing, but there in the star-filled night of communist Russia, my "enemy" was telling me, "I love you." My heart was so open the words flew out: "I love you, too."

He picked his head up and for a moment the barriers between us melted. We were eye to eye, heart to heart, soul to soul.

With the completion of his duties, he left my cabin. Immediately, I went into my knapsack and found two I LOVE YOU buttons in Russian. I pinned one on my sweater and one on my coat. I wore those buttons every day and night during my entire stay in Russia. I wanted everyone to know "I love you."

Hand and Heart

It is very difficult to separate the hand of service from the loving heart. They seem to harmonize each other perfectly. We can compensate the lack of skill in doing a service with a generous amount of love. We can also balance the absence of total love with dedicated service.

This is very much the challenge for our modern time. Some believe that it is not necessary for a doctor to love the patient as long as she or he has great skill. We are now learning that both the skill *and* the love are very important. If someone really cares about you and wants you to get well, the chances are greater for that to happen.

Hippocrates, the father of modern medicine, also seemed to believe this. When new doctors are ready to embark on their chosen service at the end of their medical education, they must repeat the Hippocratic oath. Its essence is: "Above all else, do no harm"—to do no harm to body, mind, and spirit. My suggestion to doctors and all of us in the healing profession is to start out *each* day by repeating this oath. That way the oath is a constant daily reminder that no matter what we do, "Above all else, do no harm."

I was visiting a hospital in southern India. It was early in the morning and the staff was about to change from the night to the day shift. Before seeing the patients each day, they gathered together to say a prayer for the welfare of all. Each in their own tradition, they would alternate saying a prayer for that day.

After the prayer, the team recited in unison, "Please, Lord, with all I must do today allow me to bring some relief of suffering. If I am not able to relieve suffering, at least let me not be the cause of any suffering."

By adding generous amounts of bhakti, devotion, and love to our service, miracles can happen.

Enhancing Growth

If we sow an ordinary seed, can we expect an extraordinary fruit to grow? Our ashram in rural Connecticut did not have the finest soil for growing vegetables. One day our kindergarten children went out and dug holes for planting radishes. Before putting the seeds in the ground, they stood in a circle holding the seeds tightly in their tiny fists. With eyes closed they chanted and prayed to Mother Nature to infuse the seeds with energy and make the food delicious to eat. The seeds were then interred and gently covered with soil and water. Each day the children would go out to the site and repeat the circle and prayers. When it was time to harvest the radishes, to our amazement they were three times the size of a "normal" radish. Ordinary seeds, inferior soil, but lots of devotion and love.

If this can happen with radish seeds, what then can happen to us if we give other people loving help?

·ty Begins with Love

ʾus dislike the idea of charity. In the later versions of the New
·t in the letters of Paul to the Corinthians, the word *love* is sub-
charity. Until recently it read "Faith, hope, and *charity*. And the
ʾhese is *charity*." It has now become, "Faith, hope, and *love*. And
·atest of these is *love*." In our times it seems that charity and love
have become synonymous with one another.

Sometimes the greatest service is not even knowing who or what you
are serving. We become like the sun and just shine everywhere without discrimination. The rain nourishes the crops and trees as well as pouring
water through a leaky roof. Some praise us, some blame us. We remain the
same. That is the most difficult kind of service. It is easy to say that we do
not want praise or blame for what we do, but to continue to love and serve
when things are not going our way is a true test of our conviction and dedication to service.

The yogic attribute of ahimsa (nonharming) is a powerful tool on
many levels. As we gain control over our *minds,* we are able not to cause
any harm with our *actions*. Yet it may still be difficult not to do harm with
our words or thoughts. To be kind to someone who is nice to us is easy.
Our challenge comes when we encounter those who are unintentionally
or even intentionally trying to hurt us. When we are able to control our
words and thoughts we truly receive the benefit of a peaceful heart. True
ahimsa is not doing harm, even when we *possess* the power to harm, being
kind and loving to those who are weaker or more vulnerable than we are.
The highest form of ahimsa is while not condoning others for their harmful actions to us or others, we do not hate them either. Instead we give
them love and service in return.

Mahatma Gandhi had ahimsa as one of the main principles of his life.
He brought the entire British Empire to its knees by not harming even
those who did harm to him.

My trip to Hungary was a year or so before the Russia trip, in the mid
1980s. A friend had convinced me to come to communist Hungary and
teach yoga even though it was forbidden at the time, forbidden to teach
anything that had a hint of spirit or religion. We were stopped at the
twenty-five-foot iron chain-link fence that was called the Iron Curtain. It

was sunset and the birds, circling overhead, were mocking our waiting in line at this arbitrary border.

The next days would be filled with small gatherings and talks at people's flats. For the grand finale of my stay, my hostess had arranged a "scientific" meeting at the Palace of Justice. I really wished she had not tempted fate by having this public gathering. "I want everyone to be able to come and hear you," she told me convincingly.

The day of the talk, my friend informed me that she had received a phone call from a "journalist" who wanted to have an exclusive interview with me after the talk. I was delighted until I noticed the worried look on her face. I discovered that an exclusive interview in Hungary at that time was very different than an exclusive interview in the United States. It meant that he would question me alone (with a translator) and that the questions must be answered in a certain way or trouble could be brewing. Many thought it was just another way to be questioned by the KGB (secret police). My friend was hoping to avoid this "interview" at all costs.

We arrived at the palace in time to witness the large gathering moving from the room originally assigned to us to a much larger and more impressive room. Because of the grand size of the room and the small size of me, I was asked to sit on a cloth that was placed on a large conference table so everyone would be able to see me. Both sides of the table held huge vases with fresh roses. The table just happened to be placed in front of a colossal photograph of Karl Marx. I hopped up on the table and, with benevolent disregard for "Comrade Marx" behind me, I began to speak.

It was by no means scientific, but I did try to keep it as "unspiritual" as I possibly could. I felt great. The people were with me, absorbing every word.

After a short break, I asked for questions from the audience. A small man in the front row rose to his feet to ask a question. He identified himself as a journalist (*the* journalist) and said he changed his mind and would be "happy" to let go of the exclusive interview and make it a public interview. (I later found out he meant to make it a public *humiliation!*)

The crowd started to boo. "Please, please be quiet," I begged. After a few moments, they settled down. I thanked him for his comments and said there were other people who had questions and would he mind waiting until the end? He nodded in agreement and we continued.

I formally ended the talk and invited those who wished to stay for the "interview" to please remain seated. Not one person moved. I suddenly realized that they were all staying to "protect" me—from what, I had no clue.

"Please," I said to the journalist, "ask your questions."

He stood to his full height and, with great dignity, started to insult me and tell me I was defacing his country and the Palace of Justice.

The booing was so loud I could not even hear my translator. It took me some time to comprehend what was happening.

"What have I done," I asked, "to insult you in such a way?"

"You are sitting on our altar, our altar of justice. It is a place where great men sit to make decisions for our country. You are putting yourself up like a god. I will not stand for this kind of behavior." By this time, he had really worked himself up into quite a state.

Humbly, I apologized. "I am so sorry to offend you. I sat here not to deface the altar but because I wanted everyone to be able to see me. I am a guest in your country and am not familiar with the customs." And then with a burst of inspiration to dispel the fear, I began to tell a story.

"Prime Minister and Mrs. Nikita Khrushchev visited the United States some years back, officially representing the USSR. They were invited to a state dinner at the White House. Mrs. Khrushchev, being a simple woman, was very much out of place at the formal gathering. At the end of a very fancy meal, she was presented with a small bowl of warm water with a lemon floating in it. Never having had a finger bowl, but having had lots of hot water and lemon, she picked up the cup and began to drink. Some of the other guests audibly gasped. How could she be so rude? Our First Lady, without missing a beat, picked up her cup and elegantly sipped the simple drink."

When I finished the story there was not a sound in the room. I did not realize at the time the bad feelings between the Hungarians and the Russians. Sometimes being politically naive can be a plus, sometimes a minus. After what seemed like a long pause, the crowd jumped to their feet cheering. (The time difference, I hadn't realized, was for the translation.)

Without saying so in words, they all understood that I was telling this "journalist" the preferable way to treat guests in one's country, not to publicly humiliate them for not knowing the customs.

The people in the audience all started to rush up to me, to thank me, to give me their hands in a gesture of friendship and love. One person handed me a perfect long-stemmed red rose.

As I looked through the crowd, I noticed the journalist patiently waiting his turn to speak to me. When his time came, he stepped forward with some other questions a little less hostile, but by no means nice.

Many watched and, without my consciously knowing what my hands were doing, I had one by one removed the thorns from the long-stemmed rose. When the questions were finished a pile of thorns lay at my side.

The journalist thanked me for my openness. Using both hands together in a respectful gesture, I handed him the thornless rose.

His surprise was apparent. He backed away, stunned. Making his way to one of the large vases, he took out another long-stemmed rose.

I continued speaking to others and he inched his way back to the "altar." When I saw him with the rose, I stopped my conversation and turned toward him. He offered me the rose he now held.

I graciously accepted the rose he offered from his heart. Even though it still had its thorns, it was imbued with love. The hostile anger had been transformed and was being replaced with love.

The next day as I was preparing to leave Hungary, my friend received a call from the very same "journalist" of the night before. For security reasons, he was told I had already left the country.

"Oh, I am so sorry to hear that," he said. "I was so hoping to see her again. I knew she would see me. She liked me, you know. She gave me a rose."

The path of love always seems to make us winners. Perhaps that is why Sri Swami Vivekananda's translation of the word *ahimsa* is love.

As Thyself

Yoga is the path of balance and equanimity. Sometimes as we feel the benefit of giving of ourselves, we want to do more and more. We transfer our competitive energy to the act of serving.

The Bible says, "Love thy neighbor as thy self." It seems to be necessary to learn to love and serve yourself first.

The heart, as a great pump, gives us a wonderful lesson in service. The first fresh oxygenated blood that comes into the heart is taken in and used by the heart itself. The heart doesn't say, "Oh, the stomach seems to need the blood because it is digesting right now. I'll send it there first." The heart is intuitive enough to know that it must take care of itself first. The energy-rich blood is then pumped out, feeding the rest of the body. That's a good lesson from our own hearts. Even before we help others, we must help ourselves *first*. It is only then we are inspired to work for the good of all.

The participants who came to the Commonweal Cancer Help Program varied in their disease process and prognosis. Shelly was a very fit looking out-of-doors type. She would probably be more comfortable in a jungle than on the ferry crossing San Francisco Bay.

More than four years ago she was diagnosed with a rare type of breast cancer that was identical to the one that had taken her mother's life only a short time before. She watched as her mother's life oozed out of her body over a six-month period while diligently engaging in conventional treatments. It was a painful experience and one she was not interested in repeating. When the same protocol was suggested to her, she asked if it could offer her better odds for recovery and for living well than were given to her mother. With the negative answer gripping her gut, she politely thanked the doctor and got up to leave. "When would you like to start your treatment?" the doctor asked.

"I am planning my own treatment," she replied.

With that she went directly home and phoned her travel agent.

"I have just been given six months to live and instead of suffering from the treatment I have decided to follow my lifelong dream. Book me on a trip so that I may study the wild pigs in Africa. When my time comes I want no regrets."

When I saw her *four years later,* she was on her way back to Africa for a second time, to go deeper into her study. She followed her passion and that was her "treatment" to healing.

Remembering the heart's function to feed itself first, *we* must take care of our bodies and minds so our spirit can shine through in service to others.

Even the airlines seem to agree with the idea of taking care of ourselves first. Next time you fly, *do* read the instructions in the seat pocket in front of you. It will tell you if the cabin pressure changes, an oxygen mask will appear. Place it over your nose and mouth. If you are traveling with small children, put your mask on first. This instruction is often contrary to what we would normally think to do. Isn't taking care of our children more important than taking care of ourselves? By putting our mask on first we are able to keep alert and conscious. If we lose consciousness, we could neither take care of others nor ourselves. By taking care of ourselves *first,* we are then able take care of others.

When Mother Teresa of Calcutta was asked how she was able to serve from morning to night, she said, "I get my energy from Mass in the morning and Mass at night. The rest of the day I see Jesus in everyone."

Knowing how much we have to give comes as we learn more about ourselves from the inside out, not from the opinions others have of us or how we would like to be.

As we serve others without expecting rewards, our capacity for service grows.

I loved participating in and then later leading ten-day silent yoga retreats. We would vary the daily activities. There was time for meditation, postures, breathing—all the practices that help us to know ourselves. During the day there would always be a time for service (Karma Yoga). Some days it would be working in the kitchen or cleaning the rooms, whatever needed to be done. To understand the true spirit of service many times a task was done without obvious reward. We might move logs from one side of the field to the other and back again, watching the mind in its frustration and need to accomplish. After some time the mind would let go.

The first time I participated in a retreat of this kind, I was assigned to the kitchen to wash lettuce. Slowly and meticulously I washed the lettuce with full meditative consciousness. The person in charge came by and asked if I could continue do it as perfectly but a little faster, that is, if we wanted to eat lunch that same day!

Perfection is not in the slow speed, it is doing the action at the proper time, in the appropriate way, without stress or looking for reward.

At the end of each retreat, when the silence was broken, there was a time for sharing. The retreatants and staff shared some of their experiences during the ten days of practice and silence. Most people got up to say how they enjoyed or disliked a particular part. Some were funny, some were heartwarming.

A women from the retreat raised her hand, asking to share. Coming up to the microphone, she spoke to the whole group. Looking specifically at me, she began.

"Each time the Karma Yoga period was about to begin, I hid under my bed," she confessed. "I came here as a reward for myself, a special time in my life that is only for me."

With that she continued to teach *me* about Karma Yoga.

"Eighteen years ago I gave birth to my first child. She was born with cerebral palsy and needed twenty-four-hour-a-day care. Two years later my second child was born with the same disease. My every minute was focused on the children. I had no time to think or do for myself. As life goes on we get into routines and somehow manage. Ten years ago my husband had a severe stroke, which left him paralyzed on one side. My job and time allocation increased. Five years ago, my aging mother came to live with us. I nursed her as her health deteriorated. My mother died two months ago and I gave myself this retreat as a gift."

There was not even a breath to be heard from the audience.

"So you see," she continued, "Karma Yoga, serving others, is what I understand and know how to do. I came here to learn how to take care of *me*. I hid under the bed because I was afraid that you would want me to work and I wanted to rest and rejuvenate."

Tears streamed down her face. As I looked around, I saw those tears repeated on the sea of faces. Our hearts had merged with her suffering. A healing was taking place.

"Please forgive me for not following the retreat schedule," she said.

Everyone stood and applauded and turned to hug each other. I made my way through the crowd and encircled her in my arms. Planting a kiss on her wet cheek, I said, "*Thank you* for this great lesson in service."

Taking Advantage

"What if I give to someone and they misuse it or take advantage of my good nature?"

When we give, it is not useful to bring our minds into "what if's." Be very discriminating at first as to whom you give your service. Later, when you feel more comfortable, just give. If they misuse your gift, it is their problem, not yours.

It was early morning and I was about to leave Belgrade. The threat of civil war saturated every word that was spoken. My host, a man deeply committed to peace and justice, had offered to drive me to the airport. We piled my luggage into his Volkswagen Bug and, with some chugging and sputtering, off we went.

It was a very old car and when I cautiously asked about its reliability, he assured me that it was old but very dependable.

We were on a highway about forty-five minutes from the airport when "old dependable" gave out. We managed to pull to the side of the road and safely stop.

"What will we do now?" I tried to keep my voice even. There were no signs of phones. Did Yugoslavia have something like AAA?

My escort was under the car hood, shaking his head—not a good sign.

"We will have to hitchhike," he said, taking my two heavy bags from the trunk.

"Is it safe?" I wondered if political prisoners were taken *before* a war began.

After ten minutes of trying to thumb it, a taxi pulled up. We got in and off we went to the airport. On our arrival, I offered to pay for the taxi.

"No, no, you are my guest," he said.

"We were in a very vulnerable position stranded out there on the highway," I commented. "Did the taxi driver overcharge us? He certainly *could have.*"

"He did *not* take advantage of us. If he *had* taken advantage of us in that situation, that would be his problem. Only a fool would risk his conscience to take advantage of someone in need. So much more can be gained by giving at a time like that."

I left that country, knowing that if there were more people of my friend's same moral value, the war could be averted.

Sometimes we are so afraid that we will be taken advantage of that we miss out on opportunities to give even in small ways. We rationalize other people's positions. "Why do they have to be on welfare? Let them get a job." All that we are doing in these situations is closing our own hearts. We can think that all the people are just actors, giving us an opportunity to give. As Shakespeare said, "The world is merely a stage and each must play our parts." Play them well!

I was coming out of a major department store with a friend in downtown San Francisco one Christmas and our arms were full of packages.

There was a street person begging. I reached into my pocket and offered him some money.

"Why did you give him money?" she asked.

"Because he was obviously in need," I answered, hoping that would finish the conversation.

"Don't you know that most of them are putting on an act? They really have plenty of money. They make a small fortune in begging."

I couldn't help smiling. "Would you want to have a job begging people on the street for money? If they are just acting, then consider that I just paid for a great performance."

At times like that my mother always used to quote to me, " 'There, but for the grace of God, go I.' " The more we feel we are one with all, the quote changes to "There go I."

If we just give without conditions, then our hearts are clear.

Director

When we are in great pain, the tendency is to close our hearts, recede within. That causes the emotional heart to contract, causing more pain. If we can allow that grief to transform into an opening, a giving to others, our pain is lessened. Some people are so extraordinary that even at the height of their pain they still give and are healed.

This is a story I heard on the *Oprah* show. I have forgotten the names and places but the spirit of the action stayed with me.

When Joe was called at work and told that his young wife had collapsed and was taken to the emergency room, his emotional heart imploded with pain.

Over the next weeks, she lay unconscious with a rare brain disease. She was unable to respond to outside communications. Her young children and parents came to visit, yet her physical body was unable to greet them. They continued to come as their love was still met by some unseen force.

Joe stayed by her bed day and night, pausing briefly to eat and take some catnaps in the lounge.

There, in the lounge, he made a new friend and they became bonded through their mutual grief. Missy's mother was in intensive care, her heart barely beating, kept alive by the hope of receiving a heart transplant from a donor before time ran out.

In their misery, the two shared tales and tears. Both were told the doctors had little hope for either of their loved ones to survive.

The days went on, their grief increasing proportionately with the sense of hopelessness.

The doctor was going to try one more procedure with Joe's wife, one last hope. If that failed, all was lost.

Time that day seemed to go even slower than before. The touch of Missy's hand helped to ease the endless wait.

The doctor arrived with the dreaded words, "I'm sorry. The procedure was not successful. She will not survive the day."

Joe's choked heart now erupted with the grief it was trying to confine, too massive for any one person's heart.

He "saw" his departed wife in her vibrant life, full of vigor, knowing she would never be that for him again except in his heart's memory.

At that standstill moment of grief, a message was transmitted: Allow that vibrant heart to live on. Give the gift of a healthy heart to Missy's mother.

Joe had always been opposed to being an organ donor. He and his wife, who was always in favor of organ donation, had many hours of discussion about their disagreement on this issue. But somehow, now, at this time, it seemed like the right thing to do. He offered his wife's physical heart so that another could live.

Missy's mom made a quick recovery from the transplant surgery. Now, when Joe visits, he can feel the fullness of the love emanating from the heart that now beats in the life of Missy's mom. He finds peace and deep gratitude from the gift of giving. In some small way it soothes him and his family to know that their loved one gave the gift of life to another.

How much does the person giving such a gift really live on in another person's body and life? Some interesting follow-up information from heart transplant surgery is being gathered by researchers and clinicians around the country.

People who received heart transplants started to report strange dreams and feelings about their new hearts and donors. Heart transplant information as to donor and transplant candidate is kept strictly confidential. Most hearts are shipped from long distances with little or no information about the donor.

Yet in dreams the donor would sometimes appear, asking the recipient to travel to a distant town or city, go to a specific address, and tell the family, "I am okay and I love them." The new heart recipients reported having visions of the persons who donated their hearts, confirmed by a photo in the person's home.

Is all this so strange when we consider that the heart is not just a physical pump but the hearth of our emotional bodies? Does the emotional heart really die when the body dies? As long as the emotional heart has someone to love, is it possible that it can embed itself deep within our own emotional heart? In this way we keep the love alive and the memory sacred. This allows us always to beat as one.

Sara was an extraordinary person, a joyous reflection of light in a human form. Everything she did and each person she touched was affected by that light. When I first met her, she had been teaching and inspiring yoga students for twenty years. She balanced that with being a devoted wife and mother.

Our relationship deepened even though we saw each other in person only once a year. On one yearly visit she told me that she had been diagnosed with leukemia, cancer of the blood. It had been detected on a routine physical examination.

Sara was a person who seemed to be "doing everything right." And yet we ask ourselves, "Why would *she* get cancer?" She did the yoga practices, ate a health-conscious diet, and had a great support system. We can "do everything right" and still get sick. With yoga, we inwardly search for true healing of body, mind, and spirit, not just a "cure" for our physical body. We learn to consciously heal ourselves and *live*. None of us know how long that precious time will last. We train ourselves to be fully aware and conscious when we meet life's challenges.

Yoga is not a magical practice to elude death. It is a tool to help us improve the quality of each moment, of each exquisite moment and go graciously to our merging with the infinite when our time has come. Death is the final healing, not a failure. We all are teachers and students until the last breath is returned to the earth. And many of us continue to teach and love well after the physical body is left behind.

Sara's disease progressed very slowly. She followed the cries and demands of her family to do all the recommended conventional treatments. Tortuous as they were, she kept her sweetness and smiles. We became very connected by heart and phone. She would give me detailed information, and I would support and counsel her when I could. Mostly I would just listen.

The years went on. She continued to teach and inspire others, regardless of how her body was reacting to the progression of the disease.

It was time to visit her city for my yearly workshop. When she entered the room for the seminar, I almost did not recognize her. She was jaundiced and swollen, yet her eyes, although yellow, were still filled with light.

She insisted on staying for the entire time, lying on the sofa. The last evening a group of us were going out to dinner. We conveyed the invitation, assuming she would not come. Surprisingly, she said, "Yes, I would love to come, and I would like you to meet my husband."

She tried to sip some soup and keep her heavy lids open. Her husband and I started what would turn out to be a long friendship. At the end of dinner she beckoned me close. I could feel she was burning with fever as she whispered, "I am very tired. I have done all I can. Do you think it would be okay to 'go in' now?"

"Of course," I said, "do what you need to do."

The next morning I received a call that she was in a coma.

Her husband asked, as the time was drawing near, if I would be available to perform Sara's memorial service. "I would be honored, but I must leave to do another workshop. It's on a nearby island; I could easily come back."

It seemed each time I phoned in the next few days, Sara would rally to the conscious level and we would engage in limited conversation. Her parents and children gathered from all parts of the country. All was in place, wishes granted, yet she still was holding on.

Finished with my last workshop, I was about to leave and go back to my home a thousand miles away. If I was to be there for the memorial service, some fancy manipulation would be necessary with the airlines, nonchangeable tickets and all.

"Sara, is there something more that you still need to do?" I asked her.

Silence. She was unconscious again.

Her husband picked up the phone. "I have been meaning to speak to you about starting my yoga education. Would you consider being my teacher and guiding me? I resisted all this time when Sara was teaching, and now I feel it will help me stay connected to myself and my heart."

With those words, I heard a scream. From Sara?

"That was what I was waiting for. Now I am ready to go. Will you promise to take care of him? Teach him."

"Y-y-yes." I could barely hold back the tears.

"But," she whispered, "I am not really sure how to die. Can you help me leave this worn-out body?"

I started helping her to withdraw from the body with the words, "Go to the light, Sara, go to the light." And she did.

Through "someone" rearranging the airline computers, I was able to return for her "celebration of life." So many came and spoke of how this simple beam of light had helped to guide them on their own path. It was a bittersweet celebration.

That same year Sara's husband and daughter joined me for a one-month yoga training program I was giving. Even though she was not officially registered, I felt Sara was there, too.

Loving and giving to others are gifts that continue long after the initial deed is done.

When two hearts—foreigners to each other—touch each other, they cease to beat for a moment in time. At the very next instant they start to beat in unison. To touch and embrace another allows us to feel the rhythm of our own heart.

CHAPTER 2

Thinking Makes It So—Imagery

EVEN *OBSERVING* OTHERS do a good deed affects us all.

For many of us, Mother Teresa of Calcutta exemplified the power of love. Through her dedication we are able to see that it is never too late to care, even when there are only minutes left to a life. Can we who are observers benefit by just reading about or seeing her work? This was a question posed to a group of researchers. An informal study was conducted to see if *just watching* was enough. A documentary of Mother Teresa's work was shown to a varied group of people—some were sympathetic to her; others were not. Before the video was shown, a small sample of blood was drawn from each person and immune function measured.

The entire group viewed the documentary of her work. Many of the scenes were heart opening—showing her holding and caressing premature babies, some of which were tiny and malformed. She freed a dying man who was stuck by his own blood to the street. Countless others were on wooden cots only inches apart, lined up in long rows, but they were dying with dignity because of the respect and love they were given. Of the viewers, many hearts were becoming tender. A few openly wept. Others sat with detached interest. The cynics sat with crossed arms, minds and hearts closed.

"THERE IS NOTHING GOOD OR BAD. ONLY THINKING MAKES IT SO."

—*William Shakespeare*

After the film, each participant was asked what he or she thought and felt about Mother Teresa and her work. Some wiped away tears as they said that she was a "great saint." Others said, "She was a good person, but nothing out of the ordinary." The cross-armed ones said, "She was a rogue, taking advantage of poor people."

The blood test results showed something different. No matter how the minds tried to close out the goodness and oneness with all that Mother Teresa exemplified, the imagery of seeing this great soul bring dignity to the destitute affected every one of them. Immune function had risen in all the participants.

Imagery, our inner guidance, allows us to create and experience. It is the language of the mind. The mind speaks in images and then translates those images into words. When we listen to words or concepts, we interpret them in ways we are familiar with or that we can understand.

We practice positive imagery as a means to allow the mind and body to mobilize all available resources that assist in the healing process. This creates an intention that brings about positive physiological and psychological responses, such as lowering of blood pressure, boosting of immune function, clarity of mind, calming of brain waves, decreased heart rate, production of a feeling of well-being.

Through positive mental imagery, signals are sent to the body to help it repair and sustain energy.

When asking a group of people if they do imagery, usually about one third will raise their hands. When I ask how many worry, there is laughter and all the hands fly into the air. How many of us realize that we are *constantly* doing imagery?

Worry and anxiety are examples of very powerful negative imagery that can cause great problems. When we worry we are imagining something that *could* happen. Many of us do this type of imagery all too frequently and all too well. Sometimes the results come just as we imagined or mostly they don't happen at all.

Even if the event does not occur, our bodies still produce the same physiological responses as if it did: increase of blood pressure, agitation of brain waves, secretion of adrenaline, platelets, and bile, increased heart rate, lowered immune function. Our bodies react as if the event actually happened. Just thinking makes it so.

Many of us have had the experience of arranging to meet a friend or family member at a certain time. When we arrive and they are not there, a small doubt crosses our minds. Was this the correct time and place? We wait and, as the time grows later, become more anxious. We try to phone and if there is no answer, the anxiety accelerates. The darkness comes, the rainstorm comes. (You can substitute any particular things in this part that makes you more worried, depending on how vivid your imagination is.) We begin to become engulfed in our anxiety. Of course, we each have our different thresholds of anxiety. Some would begin to imagine the worst scenarios immediately; some, within ten minutes; while others could last for twenty or even thirty minutes imagining the friend caught in traffic. A reasonable time for our rationalizations would pass and then the worry would begin. The worry thought consumes us and overpowers any positive thoughts that try to come in. How powerful negative imagery can be! Turn that same power into positive imagery and watch your life improve!

As children, we were experts at doing imagery. We would watch, listen, touch, and smell many things. We had imaginary playmates and could make dresses out of newspaper and swords out of a cardboard box. Magic and mystery thrilled us.

As our skills and bodies developed, we were then able to mimic many of these observed actions.

Even the now effortless act of walking took so much concentration and imagery to learn. As babies, we were unable to perform this act most of us now take for granted. First, we began to watch others as they walked. We watched very closely. We observed motion as we were carried. As our legs became stronger and our muscles developed, we gained the perception that they could lift and support us. Yet we were still unable to perform the physical act of walking. Through our minds and power of observation, the imagery process was slowly filtering into our body. We continued to watch and observe until one day, with the help of supporting hands from above, we were able to stand up. We were elated as well as elevated. We had conquered the greatest conscious challenge so far in our short life on the earth. And in our great moment of triumph, we might fall down—only to rise again with greater determination. Finally, one day, with constant perseverance, we were able to stand alone. The focused mind continued as we took first one step and then another, remembering, imaging. What does it look like? How would it feel? Always with great concentration, we continued to watch and study others as they walked.

When we take our first and subsequent steps, we are actually projecting an image of ourselves walking. After the image is projected by the mind, we move our physical body into that image.

A small child may be enticed to the other side of the room by holding up a favorite toy. To everyone's amazement, the child is able to walk much further and even to reach the toy. It is a movement of triumph where the child's imagery expands even beyond her own expectation, from one or two steps to the whole room and eventually the whole world.

We have all heard about or witnessed people doing unthinkably heroic feats in the face of incredible danger. How could someone actually walk into a burning building and not get burned? These heroes see themselves rushing in to save someone and bringing them out well and unharmed. They never think of the hazard of the fire. This same idea of positive, you-can-do-it imagery is used in fire walking. How could someone actually walk on hot, burning coals with bare feet and not get burned?

One of the most powerful ground rules is to focus on the goal of quickly moving out of the burning building or to image yourself on the other side of the bed of fire, well and unharmed. The mind cannot, even for one instant, allow itself to image the danger of the fire. It may seem impossible, yet many people are able to do this successfully, unharmed. It is a testament to the power of imagery. If the power of the mind is that strong, it can also help us heal.

Positive imagery allows us to accomplish goals that aid in making our lives more meaningful and productive. When we become vigilant with our practice, we receive great benefits. If, after the first few steps, the baby got frustrated and gave up, where would most of us grown-up babies be? Still crawling! Sometimes in our projecting of positive goals, we may trip over a chair or object in the way. Let it be only a temporary delay. And, like the baby, let's be sure to get up and try again with renewed determination.

Imagery relates to us in action, words, or thoughts. When we set an intention, it places a positive or negative energy charge on each thought or action. Imagery can be as simple as making plans, preparing to-do lists, or setting goals. Even in sleep, we dream. Any of these actions can be positive or negative.

Our words and verbal expressions are powerful imagery. Affirmations have become a well-known way to inspire us to positive imagery. There is an ancient yogic technique called *pratipaksha bhavana* that simply means *to cultivate the opposite.* If we are fearful and want not to feel the fear, cultivate courage. If normally critical, cultivate understanding. We begin carefully to choose words and phrases that help us to promote the positive and the negative automatically lessens.

"I am feeling strong and courageous about the meeting today." Our knees may be knocking, but our conviction is strong. After a time the positive words and thoughts will effect even our shaky knees.

When forming a positive affirmation, it is important to leave out any negative influences: "I am *not* going to eat any junk food today." When interpreting this, the mind can easily negate the *not* and the positive turns into a negative: "I *am* going to eat junk food today." It is better stated in a positive way: "All the food I eat today will be healthy and nutritious."

The softness or harshness of our speech reflects on us as well as others. It is not only *what* we say, but *how* we say it. The ancient Yogic scripture the *Bhagavad Gita* tells us how we can keep the mind calm by having *four* qualities to our speech:

TRANQUIL: Tranquil in tone and volume, without urgency or panic, having a soothing effect on others (to speak with a *velvet* tongue).

TRUTHFUL: Truthful so the heart is not blocked by confusing contradictions, saying and meaning the same thing (to speak with a *straight* tongue).

PLEASANT: The words uplift with an optimistic flow. We may even know some people who can say almost anything, even unpleasant things, and it is never taken as hurtful.

BENEFICIAL: Allow the words to have some positive effect. This could be as simple as wishing someone "good morning."

Verbal abuse is a form of negative imagery, the opposite of an affirmation. When someone is told they are stupid or ugly or they will never amount to anything, these words form a deep image on the mind that is difficult to erase—even long after the words have been proven wrong. (Keep this in mind with what we say to ourselves as well.)

An adult friend of mine related that when she was thirteen years old, an aunt came to stay with her family for a period of time. At that age many children, especially girls, seem to be all arms and legs, very gawky. My friend was quite tall for her age, and that made her even more gawky and clumsy. She bumped into furniture, dropped cups and glasses. Her knees and shins were always bruised. Her aunt constantly scolded her for being so clumsy. The visit of her aunt had passed, and after a time, grace replaced clumsiness in the girl. My friend did not see her aunt again for several years. When she did, to her surprise, the clumsiness returned. In her aunt's presence, cups were broken, shins were bumped, juice was spilled. Her aunt's mind held the image of her clumsy niece. This same embarrassing scenario was repeated with each visit. Each time they met, the aunt's image rose up to reinstate the outgrown clumsiness. Sometimes it is as difficult for us to allow others to change as it is to change ourselves!

The verbal cues we give ourselves sometimes encourage us in the opposite way. Listen to how you speak to yourself. If you are trying to slow down, it's useful to eliminate such expressions as "I'm going to run down and grab my jacket," "I'll get a quick bite to eat," or "I'm going to dash to the store." How many more can be added to this?

When we're trying to do some work, learn something new, or make a change in our lives, phrases like the following are counterproductive: "I'm so stupid," "I'll never be able to do that," "I'll never make any money doing this," and "Who would want to date me?"

All these words form images, but they are not *positive* images. Negative imagery causes stagnation in our lives and adds to the development of disease. I will often point out to my clients what they are saying. These are some of the negative affirmations I have heard over and over: "This job is eating me up alive," "My heart is broken," "My partner is causing me heartache," "He is a pain in the neck," and "She is sucking the lifeblood out of me." When they realize what they have said they are surprised, especially when it directly relates to their physical or mental health. Language is powerful imagery.

In my thirty-plus years of service with people who have life-threatening diseases, it was always important for me to see them as whole beings. In our modern medical facilities women and men are categorized by the diseases of their bodies. It is not uncommon to hear doctors, nurses, or therapists say things like "I just saw the breast tumor in 25-A" or "The amputee in 6-B needs a bedpan."

We start to think of ourselves like that: "I am a cancer patient" or "I am a heart patient." When we continually think of ourselves as patients, it is difficult to be well again. In order to get well we need to change our whole identity and identification.

The image others have of us also greatly affects our ability to heal. "Find a doctor who loves you and believes you can get well." This is a common piece of advice I give to my clients. I have heard horror stories of people given death sentences from someone "playing God." There are many people who, according to the medical establishment, should be dead, yet somehow they are still walking around healthy and strong. Many are told they will be on this or that particular medication for the rest of their life. With lifestyle changes they are able to reduce or completely eliminate the needed medication. Hope is the strongest imagery. Even in the gravest situations, there must be room for a miracle to happen.

Sometimes negative imagery comes from the religious community.

Elizabeth came to see me at a time when her breast cancer had reoccurred and metastasized to her lung. She was a very loving and proper woman who always wore a hat and gloves and carried a Bible. Her devotion to the Sacred Heart of Jesus was her strength and power. It seemed that with her present state of health and her religious openness, imagery would be a good modality for her. We practiced relaxation at each session and she was a willing student. When we included imagery with the relaxation, she had some apprehension in choosing her image. With my guidance she chose an intimate and healing image—her favorite picture of Lord Jesus in long flowing white robes, holding the Sacred Heart—it seemed to be the perfect image for her. Since we met only once a week, Elizabeth diligently practiced the relaxation and imagery techniques on her own every day. Soon she was feeling centered and experiencing more peaceful energy.

A few weeks after beginning the imagery, she arrived on time for her appointment. When I met her in the waiting room, she took my arm and ushered me into my office, closed and locked the door behind us. With light in her eyes and a giggle in her voice, she told me to sit down. "What is it, Elizabeth?" I said, now getting as excited as she.

"Well . . . ," she started too slowly for my now whirling, inquisitive mind. "I do my imagery every day like you told me to. It is usually nice, but last night when I was doing it, something happened. Instead of me just imagining the picture of Lord Jesus, he *really* appeared and then turned into *pure white light*. I could feel the light enter my body right here." (She pointed to the third eye center, between her eyebrows.) "And then I felt the light travel all through my body and this profound feeling of peace, love, and joy permeated my whole body and mind. I still feel that way even now." She carefully assessed my expression and asked, "What do you think this could mean?"

My vision was blurred with tears, the kind of tears that appear during moments of great inspiration. After taking a moment to regain my composure, I (not so cleverly) responded to her childlike wonder: "What do *you* feel it means?"

"Well," she said, "could it mean that Lord Jesus has come to me?"

Shaking my head yes was all I could do. It was a stunning moment that I shall never forget. It was, in fact, only a moment until I was snapped into a different reality.

"Elizabeth, have you told anyone *except me* about what happened?"

"No," she replied, "I came here first thing."

I had been privileged to be the first person to share with Elizabeth her very profound and positive experience. The image that had snapped me out of the moment was of a very conservative minister who might misunderstand her vision as a negative force.

"Elizabeth," I said cautiously, "it is very important that you do not tell anyone else about this. It is a very sacred healing experience and must be kept private." "Yes," she whispered, "I know." She added, "I feel like the cancer is gone." With that newfound hope, she left with the promise to return in one week.

The weekly appointment came and went. Elizabeth was not seen or heard from. Finally, after two days, I called her home. Her husband abruptly answered my inquiry and delivered a message that Elizabeth no longer needed my services.

This brought concern to me and I phoned again, hoping to reach Elizabeth directly. When her soft voice answered, I was relieved. "What happened, Elizabeth?" I asked.

"Oh," she said, "I just had to. I didn't mean to do any harm."

"What happened, Elizabeth?" I asked, even slower and softer, dreading the answer I was about to receive.

"I told my pastor. He yelled and screamed and said, 'It is the work of the devil. Not only do you have cancer of the body, you now have cancer of the soul! Never do anything like that again or you will go to hell for sure!' So I am afraid to do it again."

Perplexed, I asked if she could please come in to see me just one more time. After what seemed like a long hesitation, she softly said, "Okay."

"And be sure to bring your Bible," I said.

The next day, a very sad, broken woman named Elizabeth replaced the one I used to know. Still with hat and gloves and trusty Bible in her hand, she shyly and apprehensively entered my office.

"Elizabeth," I started gently, "how well do you know the Bible?"

"Forward and backward," she stated proudly.

I began cautiously, knowing I was skating on thin doctrine. "Do you know the part where it says, 'When thine eye becomes single . . .'?"

"Yes," she replied, " '. . . the whole body fills with light.' "

"This," I pointed to the middle of my forehead, "is called the third eye. When the two eyes draw inward from the worldly sights to the heavenly realm, they form a third eye. This eye opens to allow heavenly light to enter and then the whole body fills with light. The light, Elizabeth, was a gift from Lord Jesus."

Some of the glistening light from the land of knowing began to peek through the somewhat veiled sadness. "Oh, my, then maybe the healing light *is* from Lord Jesus after all." She was brightening by the second. "Maybe I *am* filled with healing light."

Imagery or Meditation

Meditation and imagery are different in their applications and in effect. With imagery, we are *actively creating* a situation or forming an idea. In meditation, we don't *do;* we just *are.* Meditation techniques tend to be very simple, repeating a word or phrase or observing the breath. Imagery and meditation are in the same world but on two different sides, and one very often leads to the other. I recommend doing both for maximum benefit.

Imagery or Visualization

There are different ways we image according to the way the individual mind works. To many of us imagery and visualization are the same. Visualization is using the sense of *seeing* to do imagery. Are you unable to picture things as they actually appear? For example, if I say to you, "Close your eyes and picture an apple," many of us will be able to do this because we have seen so many apples. If asked to picture an unfamiliar scene that

I described only in visual terms, you may have difficulty picturing it. However, you might be able to experience it based on your other senses. About 75 percent of us are visual imagers. The rest are a mixture of auditory, kinesthetic, or having a *sense* of the image.

All forms of imagery are valid. There is no wrong way to do it. The important thing is to find the best form for you because that is what will work best for you. Only you know what your body and mind need. If you are relaxed and open in this state of awareness, the natural intelligence of the body to heal itself will be honored.

Let's try a simple example of imagery that can help you discover which senses are most accessible to you.

(You may want to make an audiotape of this with your own voice or have someone read it to you, or listen to the *Sojourn to Healing* audiocassette from the Abundant Well-Being series. For more information on this cassette series, see the last page of this book.)

Assume a comfortable position—either lying down or seated. Allow the body to relax completely. With a relaxed body, the mind is better able to focus.

Allow the eyes to close. Take in a deep breath and let it out slowly.

Leaving the body relaxed on the floor, using the imagery of your mind, begin to stand up.

Hear your footsteps on the floor as you slowly walk out of the room. Place your hand on the doorknob, *feel* the shape and temperature of the knob. Gently turn it and open the door.

See the bright sun shining in as you open the door.

Feel the warmth of the sun on your face.

Continue to walk out into the sunlight and *feel* crisp, cool air on your cheeks.

Hear the leaves blowing in the gentle breeze. *Hear* the singing of the birds.

Smell the fragrances in the autumn air. Pair that with the sound of the rustling leaves.

See the filtered light coming through the trees.

Feel the cool, gentle wind nipping your nose.

See the beautiful green, yellow, and red changing leaves on the trees against the clear blue sky.

Look ahead and *see* a light green meadow blanketed with golden flowers.

Can you *smell* their wafting fragrance? Look beyond the meadow to a large apple orchard.

See the green trees, heavy with ripe, red apples.

Feel yourself skipping up to the trees, while kicking the piles of leaves underfoot. *Smell* the sweetness as they decompose. With great anticipation, reach up to pick a juicy, fresh apple. You are about four or five inches shy of reaching the apple. Determined, you rise up on your tip-toes, touch the apple, and the ripe apple falls into your outstretched hand.

Feel its coolness and firmness in your hand. Polish the smooth apple skin on your sleeve.

See the sun reflecting in the shining skin. Bring it up to your nose and *smell* the freshness. Touch it to your lips. *Feel* the coolness.

Open your mouth and *feel* the hardness of the apple skin as your teeth sink into the apple. Take a big bite. *Hear* the crunch.

Feel the juice in your mouth as it bursts with taste. *Taste* the sweetness of the fresh-picked apple. *Feel* the juice dripping down your chin as you chew and swallow the piece of apple.

Look up into the sky and again, *feel* the warmth of the sun.

Feel the perfection of the moment.

Slowly, with the apple still in hand, begin to walk back through the trees.

Hear the crunch of the leaves, the whisper of the wind in the trees.

Slowly come back into the room, to your relaxed body.

Bring the awareness back to the breath. Take in a few deep inhalations and become conscious of the body.

Remain still and refocus your awareness as you notice how many of the senses you used. Were you able to *see* the trees, the apple, the sun? Could you *hear* the birds, the sound of the leaves in the trees, the rustle of the leaves underfoot, the crunch of the apple? Could you *smell* the autumn leaves, the flowers, the apple? Were you able to *feel* the breeze on your face, the warmth of the sun? Could you *taste* the apple? How sweet was it? Did you actually salivate? Even though you were not physically eating the apple, your mouth and salivary glands might have reacted as if you were. Perhaps you could not tangibly engage the senses. You may have had a sense of how things were. Was there one or more of the senses that was most dominant for you? Sight? Hearing? Feeling? Tasting? Smelling?

Sensing? That one sense or a combination of senses would be best for you to focus on during your creative imagery.

If you are not a strong visual imager and wish to sharpen those skills, try this next exercise.

Sit or lie in a comfortable position with your eyes closed and imagine yourself going into your own bedroom. Begin to *see* where all the furniture is located. Where is the bed? The night tables? The dresser? Chairs?

Now go back around the room and notice the detail in pictures, photos, the color and pattern of the sheets and bedspread, the color, shape, and size of the telephone and clock, all the details that you see every day and every night.

When all that comes clear to your inner eye, move to another familiar room. Then try imagining familiar people, foods, scenes that you repeat daily. With time, begin to *see* less familiar objects and finally *see* that which you can only imagine.

Perhaps now you can better understand how powerful imagery can be in healing. If we turn our powerful senses inward, we are able to mobilize our own immune systems and healing potential—influencing our bodies, minds, emotions, and entire lives.

Using Imagery for Healing

Pain has a definite way of getting our attention. It is difficult to deny deep pain. All of our attention goes to that place. Yet in deep sleep it seems to go away or at least lessen. If we can focus our attention positively, it is possible to help any part of the body or mind to release pain and heal.

With the pain or sickness calling for our attention, we just need to meet that attention in a positive instead of a negative way. You may have a wound that is open and sore. Imagine what it looks like when it is healed. Then slowly—in your mind—create the healing.

At first this may seem unfamiliar to you. Yet the cells in your body are doing it all the time. The next time you have a cut or splinter, instead of covering it up immediately, watch how it heals. Notice that the healing comes from inside out. The immune system does its own form of imagery to heal a wound and that makes us whole again. In imagery, we are supporting the body's own natural intelligence by allowing it to have all the positive energy it needs. Every part of us is influenced by positive energy. If we are playing sports, we perform so much better if someone cheers us rather than boos us. So it is with healing.

In the community where I lived we tried our best to practice these philosophies of positive imagery and healing. One cold snowy day, I happened by an overturned sled with the seven-year-old driver tossed in the deep snow. His concerned mother was running to the scene, as was a summoned automobile, pulling up for its mission to the hospital. We carefully lifted our hurt driver into the backseat. The left arm was in an unusual position, and the pale face and quietness of the sled's pilot was alarming to us. We kept questioning him, "Are you okay? Talk to us." We remembered our basic first aid training to keep a patient conscious. With all our prompting, still no words came, but we continued to persist.

Suddenly, from the pale and quietness of the victim came the plea, "Mother, please stop bothering me. I am imagining that my arm is well and healed and that the bleeding has stopped. I need full concentration to do this. No more talking, please." A bit startled, we obeyed.

Upon reaching the hospital, we relayed the whole situation to the nurse and doctor on duty, including the part about the imagery and the need for quiet in order to concentrate fully. They respected the request with a grin, seeing it as childish play.

The grins turned into smiles when, after examining the wound, it had already begun to heal, as if the accident happened three or four days ago. "Certainly not a recent cut! Are you sure this just happened today?" the surprised doctor asked. Even the X rays revealed a normal seven-year-old arm.

The sledder's imagery had worked! His body responded to his positive and concentrated imagery.

Many people find the concept of healing energy out of the realm of their everyday life. It may take some time and practice before you are comfortable accessing this essential part of you. It often remains hidden during our busy, thought-filled days, emerging only at times of quiet or illness.

Dr. N was a gentle and brilliant research scientist. The ache in his neck was taking his much-needed vitality. After many visits to specialists, X rays and tests, prods, and pokes, without relief, it was suggested that maybe I could be of service.

We came from very different areas of health and healing. He was part of a major established medical center. I was from a place of believing that *we can* heal ourselves. I must admit I was more than a bit intimidated.

After a few words (he was a man of very few words) and some awkward silence, we began with deep relaxation. Explaining the basic principles of deep relaxation, I then asked him to access his healing energy.

"Energy?" he asked with a quizzical expression. "What do you mean by energy?

I tried several different descriptions to no avail, realizing my words were not relating the correct experience to him.

"The only energy I know is $E = mc^2$" he related to me from his vast knowledge.

I said, "I know that it is difficult to understand the concept of this subtle energy. I am not sure it is to be understood by the mind. The best way to know energy is to experience it. Will you be so kind as to humor me and pretend you know what this energy I described is? Just for this session?"

He nodded his head in acceptance of our agreement.

After our session that morning he was also at a loss for words. The energy that he actually experienced moving through him alleviated his neck pain, a neck pain that the best-intentioned physicians and treatments could not even lessen. The experience of our own healing energy speaks louder than trying to understand it with the mind.

Active and Passive Imagery

Imagery can be done in an active or passive form. Each can be used according to one's own temperament, or one form can follow the other.

In *active* imagery we formulate an action to work directly on an area in need of healing and, with concentration, we project that image to do the task.

In choosing an *active* imagery tool for yourself, it is helpful to base it on the stronger of your senses. If possible, it's good to combine the senses. For example, I may see a color and also feel its quality—as in a blue, cooling light or a warm, yellow light. A waterfall that can wash away unwanted cells can be enhanced by the sound of moving water.

In practicing *active* imagery, it is helpful to choose images you are familiar with and that you use in everyday life. For example: a delete button to purge unwanted emotions; a sponge to soak up debris; a broom to sweep away pain; a vacuum cleaner to open vessels; soap that wipes away tumors; a paintbrush to change a hot spot to a cool spot; a laser beam to dissolve blockages.

When transmitting the image to a particular part of the body or mind, it is important to be relaxed, focused, and directed. When the image gets to the area in need of healing, surround it with a chosen image and allow that part of the body to soften, open, and accept the image. Do not try to use force; instead be patient (when we are ill we are asked to *be a patient*) and allow the body to accept the healing.

In the early days of the western use of imagery, a strong, aggressive emotion was sent to "strengthen" the imagery. A cancer patient would aggressively hunt down and kill the cancer that was invading him. A heart patient would angrily root out the damaging plaque in the arteries. If you allow the image to be sent with anger or anxiety, that same negative energy may counteract the positive healing energy. You may, in fact, positively affect the particular sight you are targeting, yet the negative energy may weaken the rest of the system. The strength of the negative will win out and the action will not be of a total healing.

Did you ever have the experience of stubbing your toe? What happens? You might have been careless, not paying attention to where you were walking. We then blame the toe and say bad things to it. "Darn this toe, stop hurting." Or we insult it: "Stupid toe" or "I have a bad toe." I hear people saying that about their back: "I have a bad back." I always imagine shaking a finger at the back: "Bad back! Bad back!" That does not seem to be the best way to coax our bodies to heal.

Instead, wouldn't it be better to hold and cradle the toe, giving it love and attention? As whole beings, we respond much more to praise than blame. Love allows us to heal.

Learn to use distance and dispassion as a way to accept painful situations. A judge in a court may feel compassion for the person sentenced to death, yet she must do her duty. There can be no anger involved. If she remains calm the correct decision is made. A plumber cleans out pipes without aggression, just as part of his job. Do you think you would want a surgeon to operate on you if he came into your room yelling, "We are going to cut that [blank blank] tumor out!"? I would prefer to have someone a little less aggressive. In his heightened emotional state, I would be concerned that he would cut too much!

Anger, hatred, and fear can be the underlying causes of many of our modern-day chronic diseases. If the emotional component is not positive, it must be dealt with in ways appropriate to expression, not repression. If possible, for the period of time dedicated to imagery, stay as neutral as possible or transform the negative thoughts into positive thoughts. Sometimes when the negative becomes in control you may rid yourself of one disease yet cause another. This has been proven in and out of the laboratories many times.

Fern came to the residential retreat in a very weakened state. To walk from one building to another was difficult for her. The ovarian cancer had almost won its battle over the physical body. Bone thin and weak, she began to spend more time in meditation, withdrawing from body and mind. She drew great inner strength from the yogic practice. Within the week it manifested by producing great spiritual stamina.

Fern had a mounting feeling that she must somehow contact her ex-husband and express to him how she had felt abandoned by him. He had wandered off to his new mate in sneaky and clandestine ways, causing Fern much heartache and pain. While she lay in surgery he lay in bed with the "other woman." His vivid betrayal, especially at her time of desperate need, was becoming a perpetual image. She thought that she had put it out of her mind. Out of mind maybe, but not out of heart *or* soul.

"I have nothing to lose," she gambled. "I never really told him how I felt about the whole affair. I am going to tell him exactly what I think of what he did, in no uncertain terms. He may not like it, but you know, I did not like what he did either."

She was committed to her decision and on her departure from the retreat, the goal was clear.

The next time I saw her was one year later, I hardly recognized her. She was vital and radiant. "You look fantastic! What have you done?" I stammered. With an enormous smile, she told me the next installment of her story.

"After I left the retreat I realized that I was still very physically weak. I got the notion to go see my ex-husband in person rather than communicating over the phone or by letter. I wanted to see my home and our friends one last time before I died. I booked a flight and prayed I would be able to make it at least one way. When I arrived, my energy tank was nearly empty. I went to my former home, one I had cared for and raised my children in. There he was with his new wife. All of a sudden as if from out of the depth of me came this rage; the volcano erupted. All the anger, resentment, hurt that I had been incubating for too long finally regurgitated. Neither I nor he could believe it. I had always been the quiet, restrained one. It was a very deep pit and it spewed until the last of the lava was cooled.

"I then left, taking a few treasures of my past with me, and got on the airplane. The next weeks were spent alternating tears and laughter. Remembering his face when I erupted made me bend over with laughter.

"I began to go about my business as usual. I found that instead of growing weaker, I was gaining strength. After noticing this, I went to my doctor. His surprise found me redoing tests and scans. 'It seems the cancer is retreating,' he said in amazement."

The last time I saw her was several years later. She had moved to a new town and was pursuing her dream of a college diploma. At that time she was free of the disease that seemed to be her demise only a few years before. In her healing she was able to gain compassion for her ex-husband and his deeds. Her heart was open to healing for herself and for others.

When we hold onto things good or bad it stops the energy from flowing in and through our hearts. It can prevent healing from happening. Sometimes we need to express that pain. We may even ask for forgiveness or accept another's forgiveness. The heart opens and then we let it go. How long does it take for a disease to manifest in our bodies? Perhaps years. When applying natural methods, the healing starts with the subtle bodies—energy, mind, emotions—and then affects and changes the physical. Anytime we use the body's natural ability to heal itself, it must be a gentle and delicate process. It is not a quick or easy method. It is a process that goes beyond the body and cells to our very essence. *Natural healing takes time.*

A soft-spoken women from an upper-middle-class suburb came to see me because she was suffering from rheumatoid arthritis. She had been diagnosed with lupus erythematosus. Among the symptoms of this devastating autoimmune disease are painful flare-ups and inflammation of the joints throughout the body. During one of these flare-ups, even the smallest movement caused her intense pain. Her medication, which helped control the inflammation, had been increased, and the side effects were causing problems that added to the original symptoms.

I was unsure at first how to help this suffering, yet very loving woman. Even in her great pain she did not lash out at others. It was her creativity that showed us a way to soothe the pain.

As an artist, color spoke its own quality to her and each one had its own feeling and effect. When she arrived for her appointment, the imaginary paint box would appear. With a very soft and fine imaginary brush, I would—directed by her—paint her joints. "They are very inflamed today. They feel red. Let's paint them blue." I obediently would dip the brush in the paint and, with all gentleness and love, stroke the swollen joint. One day we tried green. "Oh, no! Quick! Take it off! Too hot," she said with a grimace. The color quickly changed, a sigh of relief was heard. When the correct colors were applied, off she would go—swelling down, pain relieved.

This may sound a bit fluffy or unreal to you. I must admit at that time I was skeptical myself. We were all convinced when the reports came in from the rheumatologist, saying that the results of her blood test that measured inflammation were showing a decrease. "Whatever you are doing," her doctor told her, "keep it up. You are doing great!"

Passive imagery acknowledges our innate ability and wisdom to heal. It allows the healing to happen with gentle and nonspecific guidance. It is done more frequently and unintentionally than active imagery, from the blessing we receive from a friend when we sneeze to the pronouncement from our doctor that we are well. When the words are said, they produce imagery that helps us feel better.

In *passive* imagery we find that our actions and thoughts are also images. Physical gestures and facial expressions are powerful forms of imagery. Sometimes we are unaware of how our nonverbal actions can be more explicit than our words. Opening your arms in an embrace at once makes anyone feel welcome. Initially, the simple handshake was a way to show that you did not have a weapon in your hand. In Japan, when bowing, the neck is exposed expressing a trust in the person, not to cut off your head!

One of the greatest imagery actions is a simple smile. It crosses all languages and country borders. It is an international passport.

If we speak words without our thoughts and actions behind them they do not have the same power.

There was a great healer who lived far out in the countryside. Coming to see her was at least a full day's journey. A mother took that journey because she felt the great healer could help her child. The child was addicted to sugar and chocolate, which was making him ill. After the long journey was accomplished, an appointment was given to the child.

Upon entering the dwelling of the healer, the mother told her of the child's problem.

"Please tell him to stop eating sugar and chocolate," the mother begged.

With a few waves of the hand the healer said, "Come back in two days."

The mother pleaded and protested, but the healer held firm. With great despondency the mother went back to her home to return two days later. This time they were immediately ushered into the receiving room. With very little formality the healer looked at the son and said, "Sugar and chocolate are not good for you. I advise you to stop eating them so that your body can heal."

The mother, although happy to hear the pronouncement, was more than slightly annoyed. She carefully asked the healer why could this not have been said before and saved them the long journey back.

The healer simply said, "Two days ago I did not have the power to tell your son to stop eating sugar and chocolate, because that was also one of my addictions. I needed to make a firm resolve and adhere to it at least two days before I could tell him to stop. Only then would my words have power."

Many times we are feeling very well. The next day, the results of our blood tests come in the mail, reporting elevated levels. Suddenly we feel ill. The only thing that changed was the report, the small piece of paper that said our tests were abnormal. That imagery could be enough to make us feel sick. The next day the lab calls, apologizing for their mistake. They posted the incorrect numbers; the results are normal. "Ahh! The blood test results say I am healthy; therefore I must be. I feel better already." All this is imagery that affects us so strongly it can manifest *well-being* or *disease*.

It is interesting that in Japan people are not told when they have cancer. Even the doctors who are patients in the hospital are not told. In the United States, we would feel indignant if information was withheld from us. I once asked a very sweet Japanese nurse why they observed this practice. What was the benefit? "We do not tell people they have cancer, because they will then picture the worst—pain, sickness, even death. Our hope is that just knowing they are ill will be enough motivation to help them become well. Mostly," she said softly, "we don't know how to tell someone they have cancer without creating a negative impression and hopelessness."

Frequently, when I work with people who have cancer, I encourage them to heal their relationships with their healthcare practitioners. They may feel angry or even abandoned by the way they were treated or told about their diagnosis. "I found a message on my answering machine last Friday night that my biopsy was positive for cancer. The message said my doctor would be on vacation for two weeks. I was frantic, angry, and hurt all at the same time. And I stayed with those feelings for two more weeks." Many are told that a particular type of cancer has a 90 percent mortality rate. How many would assume we were in that bracket? In fact, why not apply positive imagery and assume the 10 percent that survive? Positive imagery can put you in the winning top 10 percent of any class.

A great story of healing came from a dear friend who was out for a walk on a wintry day. She stopped in the library and by the time she departed, the weather had turned to freezing rain and sleet. Putting her coat over her head to protect her from the elements, she proceeded to dash across the street. The oncoming car's windows were a bit foggy and my friend's coat was gray. When the car finally stopped, Mary was down on the ground, unable to move her legs.

The confusion that followed was foggier than the windshield. Before long, Mary was in bed with her two broken legs suspended from the ceiling by pulleys. There were threats of amputation and a certainty that she would never be able to walk again without the aid of crutches.

Mary's long-term yoga practice kept her close to the knowledge that all things are possible. She understood from a deep level the necessity to keep the energy moving. She wanted to get up and stretch, to move the energy around to do the poses she so diligently practiced on a daily basis. None of this was physically possible. She allowed herself to go into a deep relaxation, asking herself the question "What would Nischala tell me to do?" The answer surfaced. "Put on a tape and imagine that you are doing all the poses." And so she did. Slowly and with concentration, she did each pose in her mind's eye. Just as she had completed her first session, *coincidentally,* I called her on the phone. Not as surprised as she could have been at my call, she laughed and told me the message she had gotten from me *before* the phone call came. She told me how great she now felt. I encouraged her to do the same imagery twice a day until she was fully recovered. The rest of the story is a happy one. She regained full use of both legs and even the slight limp that remained is now gone.

In this case Mary used passive imagery to heal her whole being, removing the injuries as well as the fear and anger from her body and mind. She could have also used active imagery followed by passive; this was of her own choosing. The important part is her mind never wavered from seeing herself walking on her own.

Through imagery, disease dissipates and health reemerges, and we feel whole and complete.

PRACTICE OF ACTIVE IMAGERY

Be relaxed in a seated or lying position and allow your eyes to close. Bring the awareness to the breath. Observe its gentle flow in and out. Use the inhalation to draw you inward to a place of stillness and peace.

You might like to equate this feeling of peace to an actual place you have been or a place you have seen or heard about. It can be at the sea, in the mountains, anywhere—in light or in darkness. It might not be a tangible place at all but just a feeling of stillness in the midst of activity, a place that allows you to let go and say "Ahhh." It is from this sacred place that the healing journey begins.

Choose a place on the physical body or in the mind that is either in pain or in some way in need of attention. The body may be seen realistically or you may see it in a more abstract manner. Slowly bring the mind to that area and observe. Why does this part need to be healed?

Keep the mind focused and observant as you slowly introduce the healing tool you have chosen. It could be your favorite colored light beam, golden sunlight, a gentle touch from a loved one. You may want to cut out the diseased part with a sharp knife or zap it with a laser. Let yourself be guided by a sense of knowing. Engage as many of the senses as you are able to make it realistic. If you are using the ocean, for instance, hear the sound, feel the power, the coolness. Whatever your image, make it clear and vital.

Never force the image. Keep the goal of healing in mind. Be patient until the area opens to this healing energy.

Allow the image to change and evolve. Listen to any subtle messages that may be given to you. (For instance, if you are using a laser beam, the color or the size of the beam may change.) Remember, there is no right or wrong way to do imagery.

Allow the image to permeate every cell for a total healing. Keep the mind fixed on this healing process for five minutes and then allow the healing energy to move out of the diseased area. Slowly allow it to flow through the entire body. Envision yourself as a whole being, not as a diseased part.

As you feel ready, bring the awareness back to the place of stillness within.

Slowly begin to observe the breath and allow the inhalation to deepen as you return to full consciousness. Observe how you feel after the active imagery.

PRACTICE OF PASSIVE IMAGERY

Assume a comfortable relaxed position. Allow your eyes to close. Bring the awareness to the breath. Observe it gently flowing in and out. Use the inhalation to draw you inward to a place of stillness and peace.

From that place of stillness, encourage the healing energy to move through the body and the mind in the form of light, color, or just a feeling. This energy will allow the creation of a balance that brings health and wholeness. Observe how this energy seeks out and embraces specific areas. Notice how the energy permeates each cell and is welcomed. Listen and observe any messages that may be given and how that healing energy makes that part of the body feel.

Allow the healing energy to slowly expand and embrace the entire body, infusing each organ and cell in the body. Observe as the healing energy slowly infuses each thought in the mind.

Observe the feeling of peace and wholeness.

Expand the healing energy as it moves past the periphery of your own body to engulf and cushion you in healing energy.

Slowly and gently return to the stillness within, the wellspring of healing energy. Observe the gentle breath and gradually deepen the inhalation as it brings you back to the present. Observe how you feel.

"THE HEART HAS

ITS REASONS

WHICH REASON

KNOWS

NOTHING OF."

—*Blaise Pascal*

CHAPTER 3

Deep Rest, Deep Relaxation

"ANY FOOL CAN BE

FUSSY AND RID

HIMSELF OF

ENERGY ALL OVER

THE PLACE, BUT HE

HAS TO HAVE

SOMETHING IN

HIM BEFORE HE

CAN SETTLE DOWN

TO DO NOTHING."

—J. B. Priestley

THE GREAT IMPRESSIONIST PAINTER Claude Monet was sitting on a bench, overlooking his prized lily pond. It was a glorious day, with sunbeams dancing among the lilies. A friend approached Monet. "Ah, resting on such a beautiful afternoon?"

Monet, with eyes half closed, looked up and replied, "No, working!"

Later that day, the same friend again saw Monet, this time at his canvas. "Humm, now you are working?"

"No," said the painter, "now I am resting!"

There are as many ways to relax as there are people. We each have our own way of letting go of the tensions of everyday life. Some of the ways are productive, some are less productive, and some are actually harmful.

We may choose to take a walk, a nap, a warm bath or listen to some soothing music. The deeper the level of relaxation, the more lasting the effects.

With our busy lives, for most of us, relaxation is not a priority. When I ask people in yoga classes what they do to relax, a common answer is our contemporary types of "relaxation"—watching TV, competitive and spectator sports events, walking, reading, and so on. If we could measure brain waves, heart rate, and pulse rate while reading the newspaper, what would that look like? Imagine if the stock market went down, or the construction of a nuclear power plant was planned near your home, or your favorite sports team lost. Relaxing results would not appear on the tools of measurement. These forms of relaxation may have some beneficial effects, but they may not be able to produce the rejuvenating effects of a real deep relaxation.

Usually what we *call* relaxation is shifting our ordinary thoughts to another set of thoughts—often mindless activity. It is sometimes appropriately termed "killing time" or "wasting time." For most of us, that is neither conducive to productive activity nor to relaxation.

In deep relaxation, there is a physical softening of our bodies and a sense of distancing and detachment from our problems and worries. Tension melts away and thoughts surface as air bubbles escaping from the bottom of a muddy pond. There is a pop and a release when they merge with our conscious mind.

I was involved in private practice at a holistic health clinic where health practitioners from different disciplines observed various aspects of patients' bodies and minds to help them heal, to become whole. My part was using the ancient techniques of Yoga to aid them in healing themselves. Many of my clients at that time were coming for relief from chronic pain, hypertension, autoimmune diseases, and cancer.

Very often I would see patients referred by other practitioners who did not have any further treatments to offer. I had a small, windowless office with a tiny desk. The main piece of furniture in the room was a very large well-padded brown velour lounging chair, lovingly called the "womb." When a tense, painful body reclined with feet up and head back in this "womb," the famous and familiar sound *"Ahhhh"* would resonate through the room and through time.

The big, the strong, the tense, the proper—all would succumb to the nurturing properties this chair represented. The physical relaxation had begun. To my amazement, some of the patients were so stiff and tense that they would hover over the chair. As the sessions progressed, they would sink deeper and deeper into the cushions and themselves.

The art of deep, complete relaxation is one of the safest and most effective ways to manage stress, relieve pain, regain and maintain health, and attain peace of mind. Many have reported that their sleep became deeper, and if they awakened in the middle of the night with anxiety (50 percent of Americans report doing just that), these simple techniques allowed them to return to a deep sleep more quickly (see Chapter 8, Prelude to Sleep).

This might seem like a strong claim for something so pleasant to do, but the proof is in the doing.

The calmness of the body then leads to calmness of the mind. When the mind calms, it sees thoughts like separate frames on a filmstrip. Seeing the thoughts individually allows our reaction time to lengthen, giving us that needed time to make choices consciously rather than to react automatically.

One of the ways this is accomplished is through the relationship of deep relaxation to the peripheral nervous system and its two components, the sympathetic and parasympathetic nervous systems. Simply stated, the sympathetic system tries to insulate us from danger by giving us a surge of energy to fight or flee. If we are threatened or imagine we are threatened—even by doing something like taking a written test or being asked to give a speech—this system gives us sympathy by supplying us much-needed energy in the form of adrenaline to get away and fast. This energy surges to our hearts and our extremities. Our pupils dilate so we can see better and we have the ability to dash quicker than an Olympic athlete. We have heard cases of mothers doing extraordinary feats to save a child. Their bodies and nervous systems sympathized with their need to act quickly and heroically.

After a stressful activity, the appropriate reaction would be to let go and relax. Most of us these days disregard the parasympathetic system's need to take over. We just keep going from one stressful situation to another. Can you imagine what would happen if we used our cars like we use our bodies? Using the accelerator and the horn but not the brake pedal would be a real disaster!

Both of these components have a specific function with the organs of the body. Using the heart as an example, the sympathetic aspect allows the heart to squeeze and beat; the parasympathetic aspect allows the heart to rest. They make a great team. One coaxes the heart to squeeze and the other to rest, a perfect balance.

The heart in its simple form starts to beat and pump blood sometime during the first two months of your stay in the womb, and it continues until the final beat, sometime near the last exhalation. It beats continuously without rest. It is not like the stomach that rests at night when its job is done (hopefully!). The only time the heart rests is between beats. That is *one* reason to keep the parasympathetic nervous system strong and healthy. It allows the heart its well-deserved rest.

To further understand that relationship, look at the measurement of blood pressure. The top number, or the systolic, is controlled by the sympathetic nervous system, and the bottom number, or the diastolic, is controlled by the parasympathetic nervous system. Let's use 120/80 as an example of a "normal" blood pressure. Your doctor might be concerned if your blood pressure was 180/90, but more concerned if it was 160/100. In the latter, the message you are being given is that your heart is not *resting*. I have worked with many people who were told they would need to be on blood pressure medication for the rest of their lives. They found with regular practice of deep relaxation, their blood pressure was lowered and they were able to stop taking their medication. And if deep relaxation is done continuously, it can be *brought down to stay*.

Another aspect of the heart is that, on an emotional level, it is like a revolving door: It takes in and gives out. When the heart is in the open *out* position, we *give out* love and compassion. In the open *in* position we *take in* love and compassion. Problems come when the heart ceases to revolve. If it stays open *or* closed we become stuck, not able to give or receive. It is an unnatural position for the heart. If it stays in one position too long, physical and emotional disease can occur.

Learning to relax is similar to any other practice that we want to do well. Learning to dance or play a musical instrument takes time, interest, and a lot of practice. So it is with relaxation. Most of us are not given instruction or explained the value of how or why we need to take the time to relax. I find it quite interesting that, with all the many wonderful and important things we learn in school, relaxation is stunted at our kindergarten graduation.

Deep relaxation, when practiced regularly, allows us to become aware of how quiet and still the body and mind can be, transposing that awareness into our active, daily life. We begin to notice how we use the body and how to prevent the tension from building up or accumulating. After a while, the relaxed state becomes the norm and tension is the stranger that invades our life.

With all this, our lives become more enjoyable and fulfilled. We are then able to open our hearts to embrace the wonders and beauties surrounding us—to feel that we are not separate but an essential part of the one creation.

When I began teaching yoga in 1974, it always inspired me to see that in the cycle of even one class (one hour and fifteen minutes) students seemed to let go, melt into the floor. Their bodies seemed to lengthen and soften. Their faces became younger. The groups then were in their twenties and thirties—stressed, yet still full of regenerating power.

Now the students look different. The stress is thicker, like a suit of armor, difficult to shed, acting like a second skin. It's so much like a second skin that people do not realize they are wearing the stress.

In the early years of The Lifestyle Heart Trial, the importance of deep relaxation was evident. The class initially included a relaxation only at the end, after the postures. After adjusting and adapting the practices to an older, sicker, and more stressed population, a relaxation was added in the beginning as well as after the poses. The results were that the stretches were done with more ease, and when it came to the long relaxation at the end, it was deeper. Many have reported to me that initially relaxation was the most difficult part, but after a while it became the most liked part. That is the way I teach even today, and I observe that people can stretch and bend better when they relax first.

THE FIVE BODIES AND FIVE STAGES OF RELAXATION

There are many different techniques of relaxation available in our modern times—all with good value. The one I offer here comes from the *Yoga Sutras of Patanjali*. This technique is called *pratyahara,* meaning "withdrawal of the senses." The classic example that is given is of the tortoise who is able to withdraw its limbs into itself to retreat from the world.

If I walk into a room with a sad face, you might ask me how I am feeling. When I answer, "Fine," you might think, *You sure don't look fine!* Instead of looking at my physical face and body, you are in fact looking at the reflection of my mind. My body still looks like a body with its limbs, trunk, and organs. The face still has a nose, eyes, ears, mouth. But somehow the shoulders are slumped, the back rounded. The corners of the mouth are curled down. The eyes, being the reflection of the mind and soul, have a sadness to them. The thoughts of the mind are projected onto the body like a film projected onto a screen. Even if you are unable to "see" my sadness, you might be able to feel it when I enter the room. We are multidimensional beings—beings of body, mind, and spirit.

To relax the body and mind fully and deeply, they must be temporarily relieved of their duties. All the muscles in the body must be allowed to let go, knowing that the body will be totally supported. The mind is also given this time to let go and relax. This is not a time to think of what needs to be done; instead the body and mind are given a mini vacation.

According to traditional Yoga texts these coverings, or bodies, are called *Maya Koshas,* literally, *maya* (illusion) and *kosha* (body or sheath). There are five of these "bodies" covering the pure self or the light within. Our inner light is the only constant that does not change. Everything else, like the nature surrounding us, is illusory because it is in constant change.

It is necessary to relax each body or sheath systematically from the outer to the innermost part of us for complete healing to take place. It is helpful to know what to expect in the five different stages of relaxation. Experiencing only one or two stages at the beginning of the practice is common. Allow one to lead you into the other and deeper into relaxation. It is like a labyrinth: You enter from the outside (the outer circle) and as you wind back and forth, deeper and deeper, you may be drawn back to the outside world by a sound or a physical sensation, only to retreat back inside. As you continue, you wind your way to the center where peace is finally felt. The journey back begins, and when you return to the outside, you are somehow changed, more relaxed, aware in the everyday world.

The Physical Body

In Sanskrit the "sheath" known as the physical body is called *Anna Maya Kosha,* or the body of food, what we would usually call *the body.* This is the body made up of bones, muscles, organs, blood—all wrapped up nicely in a bag of skin, decorated with hair and nails. The soybeans you ate yesterday become the teeth and hair of tomorrow. The physical body is stressed and affected by posture, temperature changes, repetitive movements, and the food and beverages we consume. We typically do not notice our physical bodies unless they hurt or we sit or lie still. At this time they whisper or scream messages of how they feel. Much of the time, we tend to ignore them and after a night's rest, we return to our good *and* bad habits. As stress accumulates, the bodily feelings it produces are accepted as a normal part of life. Getting older becomes synonymous with aching and stiffness.

By learning how to relax and release tension from the physical body, the suppleness returns, and with it, a feeling of youthfulness.

Much of our day we ignore the condition of our physical body. Sometimes, as we become more adept at relaxation, just a simple thought, observation, or awareness of the body will trigger the relaxation.

In order to relax a chronically tensed muscle, we stretch it out and make it even tighter than it already is. Exaggerating the movement in the direction of the tension helps it to relax. It's along the same lines as fighting fire with fire. We release tension using tension. Consciously tighten the body to relax it. Have the stretch be even and balanced—all the parts should feel equal. Isolate the part being stretched from the rest of the body, keeping all the other muscles in the body relaxed. First, we notice where our tension is stored, then by squeezing, we coax it to let go. This is an important observation, because during our busy days, we are less observant and stress our bodies in the ways we use them.

In this first stage of relaxation the energy moves upward from the external limbs. As we withdraw the energy from the legs we temporarily disconnect from the earth's gravity to go more deeply inward.

Do you spend a large part of your day either standing or walking? By stretching the legs out all the way from the toes to the hips, you can observe where the legs might be tight or sore. Is the inside or back of the leg tighter? Sometimes one leg is favored. Do you drive your car mostly with one leg? Is that the leg that feels tight now? By doing relaxation regularly the consciousness of how we use the body increases. When we are able to balance the energy *in* our legs, we are able to balance *on* our legs and that physical balance gives us stability in *everything* we do.

Our legs directly affect the lower back. When there is strain or tension in one or both legs, the lower back feels tense. The reverse is also true. Notice as you move and relax the legs that the lower back also relaxes. Sitting all day in chairs with our legs crossed causes quite a bit of low back distress and cuts off the circulation to the legs and feet, sometimes causing them to swell. Notice how you sit in a chair. Are you sitting up straight or are you compressing your lower back and sacrum? The one who named the base of the spine sacrum thought something *sacred* was stored in there! Yogis believe that within the sacrum is the storehouse of our energy (Kundalini). When we sit on it, we restrict the upward movement. Sitting erect allows the energy to move.

In Asian countries there is much less low back pain. One of the reasons is that people rarely sit in chairs. One day I was shopping at a major department store in San Francisco, where there is a very large Asian population. As I rounded a rack of clothes, I nearly collided with a gentle middle-aged woman squatting on the floor. She smiled and said she was shopping with her daughter and got tired, so she just squatted to rest and relax her back. It seemed to me a very sensible way to rest. Most of us would not be comfortable sitting or squatting on the floor of a public place. It is neither comfortable for our western bodies or for our social acceptability.

As we relax the hands and arms, we realize the tension that is caused as the result of carrying a purse, a briefcase, packages, or even playing tennis or golf. Any repetitive movement or strain on the wrist, elbow, or arm can cause imbalance, especially if it is a unilateral sport. Carpal tunnel syndrome is becoming more and more common as we keep our arms still and let our fingers do computer work.

Stretching out the hands and the fingers, we notice how they go into five different directions. How much space is there between each finger and the bones in the hand? How far back can you stretch the fingers? Most of us have our hands chronically gripping or in fists. Ready to fight? Holding on? How does it feel to consciously make the hand into a fist? Notice how the hand and the wrist and then the forearm begin to tighten and that tightening goes all the way up to the elbow, upper arm, and into the shoulder and shoulder blade. Could clenched fists be one of the reasons we have chronically tight shoulders in our society?

Become aware during the day if the hands are curled into a fist or gently relaxed. When we turn the palms up so the hands are open, we are placing them in a receiving position. This makes us feel mentally receptive. Because of our daily posture and habits, our shoulders and chests are caving inward. We carry great burdens on our shoulders, protecting our hearts against hurts—new or old—and harboring old emotional wounds. This makes us look older and more weary. Allowing the palms to face up helps to rotate the shoulders and chest outward, relaxing them, while opening to receive.

The abdomen is both the covering and protection for the soft and vulnerable vital organs. Notice that the abdomen extends from the pelvic bone to the bottom of the breastbone. Even though the fashions today call for a tight abdomen, it should come from muscle tone rather than trying to hold the belly in. The belly must be relaxed in order for the breath to flow easily in and out. (More about the breath later.) Tension and fear dictate a holding and hardening of the belly. When we relax the belly, we often do it with a rush of air from the mouth: "ahhhh!" The abdomen relaxes and softens, letting go of tension.

Beneath that strong housing of the ribs and the muscles are the delicate lungs and heart. With the inhalation the chest, ribs, and muscles expand; the lungs fill and balloon outward. With the exhalation, the chest ribs, muscles, and lungs let go and move more freely and the breath becomes smooth and gentle.

Most of our shoulders are chronically tensed. Typically they are up near our ears. Many of us these days seem to "shoulder" too many responsibilities. How many of us carry heavy shoulder bags or hold the phone between our neck and shoulder, sometimes for hours at a time? If we can let the burdens go from our shoulders, we will look and feel more relaxed and happy.

Notice how much energy is needed to keep us upright. Whether sitting or standing, we are resisting the natural downward pull of gravity. The back and spine carry much of this burden and are all too often the recipient of aches and pains.

The neck is a great place for tension to get caught as thoughts and feelings make their way from the head to the heart and from the heart to the head. Physical and mental tension in the neck may manifest as stiffness and headaches.

The face is a reflection of our minds. When we observe the face closely, we can see joy, anxiety, and sorrow etched into it. Look at yourself in the mirror after a difficult day. Compare it to the photos on your summer vacation. An open face and sparkling eyes express vitality, regardless of chronological age. No amount of cosmetics can change the tension reflected in the face. Notice if your face feels and looks smooth and relaxed or tense and hard. What does the looking glass say to you? Are you relaxed or fatigued?

Do you clench your jaw when you are tense and perhaps even grind your teeth at night, causing more tension? What happens to the rest of the face when the jaw is clenched? When the jaw and lips are slightly open and relaxed, doesn't the face and even the mind feel more relaxed? If the jaw is relaxed and the lips are slightly apart, a slight coolness can be felt on the inside of the lips and teeth.

The sense organs and especially our eyes are the main resources for routing information from the outside to our inner world. So much time is spent with our eyes focused and fixed on watching TV, working at computers, reading, driving, and so on. Allowing the eyes to be soft and relaxed is a way to keep the vision clear and eliminate eyestrain. The worry lines engraved on our forehead can be erased by an imaginary hand soothing away all tension and worries.

Through squeezing and relaxing each body part we can free up the energy in the physical body. In this way we liberate ourselves from the restraints of the physical body. When the physical body relaxes, a feeling of heaviness is felt.

The Energy Body

The next "sheath" is the *Prana Maya Kosha,* the body of energy, *prana* or also known as *chi* or *qi.* We perceive this energy as the physical body's aura or force field, enabling it to function and move. Even the most expensive, high-powered automobile will not be able to go anywhere without fuel; the same goes for our physical vehicles. This *prana* feeds the *physical body* and the *mind.*

Do you make efficient use of your energy? Do you need stimulants—coffee, tea, chocolate, sugar—to get you through the day? Do you have fuel to spare or do you use the last bit, leaving you tired at the end of the day? Do you ever use the expressions "I have no energy" or "I am exhausted"?

This energy body is very subtle. In its subtlety it is very powerful. Since this body does not have muscles and bones, we must look a little differently to find its anatomy and physiology. The movement of energy is seen outwardly as the breath. When we breathe, along with air we take in *prana,* vital life force. Air is distributed to all parts of the body by the breath. *Prana* penetrates into the spaces between and within the cells, organs, and bones. With gentle guidance from the mind, we use the breath deliberately to infuse the cells with vital energy and invite the tension and discomfort in the body to melt away.

Sometimes, as I am guiding this stage of deep relaxation, I will use the words "Inhale, and, on the exhalation, send the breath out through the toes." Invariably, someone who was listening very closely will say to me, "How can my toes breathe? The air cannot get out." If we think of our bodies as solid, fixed objects, nothing can move either in or out. Yet we know that even in a very solid-looking object there is space between cells. Did you ever look at a piece of skin placed under a microscope? There are wide-open spaces between the cells. Could *prana* be lurking there? In our mind's eye, when we breathe, relaxing energy into the toes, it replaces and releases tension, creating more space. It is similar to lubricating a car: When we squeeze new grease in, the old grease comes out automatically. When we send fresh vital energy into and between the cells, the tension that was there before gets squeezed out. The effect: We feel more relaxed!

Through the energy body we experience the power of the intentional breath. By taking deep full inhalations, the full exhalation that follows has the power to release stress.

As the breath is directed down through the legs and out through the tips of the toes it has the ability to release tension in the muscles, bones, ligaments, and nerves in the legs and feet. The same process is done with the fingers, hands, and arms up to the shoulders. The breath acts like water, meandering down the legs and dripping off the toes, taking tension with it. When the limbs are fully able to relax, they become heavy and weigh the rest of the body down like anchors. The result is the body becomes very heavy and still, allowing it to relax easily.

With the same process we observe the front of the body becoming soft and yielding. The back and spine let go of tension as they melt into the floor with relaxation.

The intentional breath softens all the lines and holdings in the face. Like the smooth face of a baby, worry-free, contentment emerges.

The balanced breath and energy when directed to the mind slows all the movement of the thoughts in the mind. The mind becomes calm.

The surrendering effects of relaxing the physical body are enhanced by accessing the energy body. The entire body becomes very heavy—like a small child asleep, abandoned to the cares of the world. When you lift a sleeping child, surrendered to a restful sleep, notice how heavy he feels. As adults, even in deep sleep, it is difficult for us to achieve this total relaxation. Is it any wonder that as children we awaken filled with energy both in the morning and after naptime? When we are able to relax like children, we may also have the same boundless energy in our waking state.

We experience a letting go of tension and become more relaxed on both the physical and the energetic levels. As the energy withdraws to the more subtle bodies, the physical body becomes heavy. It may feel like it weighs one thousand pounds. Being a new experience, at first the heaviness may feel uncomfortable. After a short time the enjoyment of the relaxation will outweigh any feeling of discomfort.

Once we can let go of the physical holdings on the body, we can begin to relax the next "body," or sheath.

The Body of the Mind and Senses

The next "sheath" is the *Mano Maya Kosha,* the body of the mind and senses, where our everyday thoughts and feelings reside. In this body we store everything we have learned and perceived, all our sensual perceptions, spelling, math, likes, and dislikes. Many times, the physical body is tired and wants to take a rest or siesta. The mind may intervene: "Don't sleep. Work needs to be done. Have a cup of coffee or tea instead and keep working."

To access this "body" we call once again on the breath. This time, it is the gentle, natural breath. The mind directs the gentle breath to different parts of the mind-body where we store our thoughts, memories, pains, and hurts. Each time we are injured—physically, emotionally, or with words—scars form. These scars remain in this mind-body. You may have experienced accidentally cutting your finger as you were slicing an apple. Long after the physical body healed the wound, you may have protected that finger. A *physical* scar may remain to remind you of the injury. There is an *emotional* scar also.

We have all heard tales of the phantom limb syndrome. It has been medically documented and acknowledged. A part of the physical body—an arm, leg, finger—is removed surgically, yet the person still has aches and pains where the body part used to be. There is no physical part still connected to the physical body to feel pain. Where, then, *is* the pain? The pain is in the memory of the subtle body of the mind and senses.

When relaxation penetrates the body, scars are soothed and the injuries in the physical and subtle bodies are encouraged to heal. In this stage of relaxation you may experience different thoughts and feelings emerging and surfacing. They are being released from deep within. All you have to do is stay relaxed and let them pass.

A dear friend of mine was feeling a bit queasy. Being the mother of four children, she suspected she might be pregnant again. After a few days, she became comfortable with the familiar memories her body had stored. Wanting a medical confirmation, she went to her longtime obstetrician. After examining her, he said, "No, you're not pregnant. It's probably just the flu or fatigue." Even the chemical testing did not show a positive result.

When she returned from the appointment and told us the results, we all laughed. Why would she accept the opinion of another person—even if he has extensive training and book learning—over her knowledge about her own body? Her inner experience and remembrance knew what she was experiencing on a cellular level. She needed to trust herself. Eight months later, her fifth child was born.

The heaviness of the physical body, which we felt in the previous two stages of deep relaxation, is replaced with a feeling of lightness, an almost floating sensation. I have actually seen students whose arms or legs float up and only after they have come back to physical consciousness do the limbs come back to the ground—sometimes to the student's great surprise—with a thump.

It is interesting to observe the movement of the mind and thoughts as they meander through a still body. The breath is seen clearly as the tangible link that reflects relaxation upon the body, then the mind.

It is interesting to note in yourself which part of the body feels the lightness first and which part may be more reluctant to move to the next stage. It is sometimes enlightening to question or investigate the reasons why there is heaviness, pain, or even disease in a particular area. Is more tension held there because of posture, work-related movements, or perhaps even some emotional reason? As the neck is the highway between head and heart, sometimes there may be a roadblock in the neck. If a conflict arises between our thoughts and our feelings, this can cause neck pain. Obstacles that inhibit the movement of the breath can teach us a great deal about how we think and feel.

In stressful situations, the breath comes in quickly and stays shallow. We then tend to hold the breath and tighten the abdomen. As we learn to relax deeply, the expansion of the chest and abdomen becomes slower and fuller. A prolonged exhalation encourages us to relax and release. This enhances a feeling of "taking your time" and completely letting go. The inhalation and exhalation are in a natural rhythm with each other. Our thoughts and emotions follow the same pathways.

The gentle breath can be directed to remove any subtle tension, thoughts, memories, or injuries from the feet and legs. All those times you hurt and skinned your knee as a child can be released along with all the feelings of foolishness and failure at having fallen or missed the goal.

As you direct the gentle breath to the hands and arms, can you let go of all of those feelings you are holding onto? Sometimes it seems as if our lives are a long roller-coaster ride and we are *holding on* for dear life. Ask yourself who or what you are carrying on your tight shoulders.

Did you have any injuries or operations in the pelvic area or belly? The mental scars are able to be healed on this subtle level. We hold so much in our bellies that we need to release thoughts and feelings on a regular basis.

Our chest and lungs may be holding sorrows and sadness. As we embrace the heart with healing energy it is able to free itself of emotional pain and heartaches. The throat dissipates any words that we are unable or afraid to say. When the front of the body feels soft and light, the thoughts or images have been emancipated from the *mano kosha.*

Many of the surgeries done to alleviate back pain are unsuccessful. Could this be because the pain is not *just* in the physical body? How much of our back pain is from muscle and nerve pain, and how much is from the thoughts we hold? The gentle breath can release thoughts or feelings from the entire back and spine. Sometimes we tuck some longtime sorrows or heartaches in between the shoulder blades and behind the heart. Another great storage place thoughts or feelings get stuck is in the neck. Liberating them allows the heart and head once again to resume their dialogue.

What story does your face tell? Are you able to observe a contentment in your face? Are the jaw and mouth telling a tale of tension? Do the eyes soften as they release unpleasant sights? Do the trophies of worry on your forehead remind you of repeated events?

As we let go of our emotional holdings in the entire mind-body we feel lighter.

The Body of Higher Wisdom

The next "sheath" is the *Vijnana Maya Kosha,* the body of higher wisdom. We all have that higher wisdom inside us, sometimes called intuition or knowing.

Accessing it and getting to trust it is the difficult part. We go to others or rely on books to tell us what to think, feel, and even how to heal ourselves.

It is not unusual to find that when we relax the body and mind, the greater knowledge from within comes to the surface. Some people have gotten great messages about themselves and their healing from going deep within.

Gail, a woman I knew, was using the practice of deep relaxation to mobilize the deep healing inside to help her immune system "defeat" the foreign invasion that had taken over her body—cancer. Dutifully and lovingly she would take thirty minutes twice each day to relax. One day, during the relaxation time, she kept hearing a word. The word then became a name, a name with the initials M.D. after it. The name stayed even after she came back to consciousness. Not really believing that messages could come out of just relaxing, Gail went on about her day. She kept hearing the name in her head. Checking the local phone book, to her shock and amazement, she found the doctor's name and phone number. Her hand shook as she dialed the phone.

"Doctor's office," was the response on the other end. "May I help you?"

Gail hesitated and then said, "I know this sounds crazy, but . . ." and she told her story. After a longer period of silence than Gail felt comfortable with, the nurse told her that Dr.———just last week had discovered a new treatment for the particular type of cancer she had. "Would you like to make an appointment?"

Freed from the relaxed body, we begin to feel a sense of lightness, a weightlessness. We observe a distancing and detachment from the intellect, the senses, thoughts, and feelings. The mind becomes like a crystal, reflecting clearly what we see without coloring it with our likes and dislikes, our prejudices, even our hopes and dreams. There is a serenity, an almost stillness to the breath. This awareness offers us a rare form of energy—one that is not concerned with appearances or things to do. We are open to our higher knowledge.

The *prana,* which is no longer needed to move the body or the thoughts, can be stored. Little energy is needed and little energy is used. Your *pranic* bank account is full. This is the experience of the *Vijnana Maya Kosha,* the body of knowing.

The Body of Joy

The next "sheath" is called the *Ananda Maya Kosha,* the body of joy. We go to that state of stillness, peace, bliss that we all know exists deep within each of us. Here we taste the reflection of our true self.

Perhaps we have touched this stillness while gazing at a sunset or looking into the eyes of a newborn baby—a merging in the flash of a moment. Poets and sages have written about this intimacy for thousands of years. Yet most of us do not allow for the time it takes to nourish it. As we know comfort and contentment, a feeling of being centered, we are able to surrender to that inner stillness. We savor that stillness without the sensation of body, breath, or thoughts. Here we find an endless well-spring of energy. Our deepest healing emerges, cradled by the peace of our own true nature.

The Return Trip

Bringing the consciousness back to the body and mind at the end of a deep relaxation can be as important as the relaxation itself. It is necessary to be gentle, integrating all the relaxed parts back together. We experience the energy entering with the breath and awakening all the bodies. They are all recharged with fresh, vital energy. Awaken the physical body by sending the energy first to the vital systems and then to the extremities. The slower we are awakened, the better we are able to integrate the bodies and the relaxation effect.

Occasionally, when we get close to that deep, still state of relaxation, a fear might come. Perhaps we are going to lose our identity! We may even take a short journey out of the physical body and fear we will not have a way back in. Leaving the body is not so unusual. We all do it at night in dreams. Often we are jolted back in by the alarm clock. Most of the time, we are without awareness that we have been out and about.

To help alleviate anxiety around these journeys, taking in a few deep inhalations will find you right back in your body and back in control.

How did you feel *before* and how do you feel *after* a deep relaxation? The energy affects the body, which in turn affects the mind, which impacts how we live our lives.

Staying Awake

Deep relaxation takes place in the window between the wakefulness of activity and the unconsciousness of sleep. It is a *conscious* process with full awareness at every level. Only during wakefulness can we realize the full effect and the healing benefits. Some people report that after listening to my audiocassettes for one year or longer, they still hear new words each day. This makes me very suspicious, so I include some hints for staying awake during relaxation.

If you hear someone snoring, *it could be you!* Snoring is a sure sign that you have fallen asleep. If this happens in the beginning of your practice, it is because you are probably very tired. See if you can get more sleep— but not at the time of conscious relaxation practice.

If you continue to sleep during relaxation, check with your doctor and see if you are taking too much medication—that includes coffee and other stimulants that might not let you get a deep sleep at *night*.

Tips for staying awake:

Practice deep relaxation on the floor or in a chair rather than in your bed. The sleep vibration is firmly embedded in the mattress.

Choose a time when you are fully awake (for instance, in the morning rather than at night).

Keep one of your arms bent at the elbow so that the forearm and hand are raised. When you start to fall asleep, the arm will relax and the movement will usually awaken you. If not, the arm will touch your abdomen and that will usually wake you up.

Keep one muscle group tight—for example, your thumb and first finger touching. You can do this in conjunction with the previous suggestion.

Keep your eyes half or fully open. Allow them to be still, not move
  around. When you begin to fall asleep, the eyes will start to close
  and you can catch yourself and wake up. (Most people cannot sleep
  with their eyes open.)

Sit up in a chair.

If all of this fails, you must really need the sleep. Enjoy!

Setting the Stage for Relaxation

Before you begin the practice of relaxation, be sure that you will not be
disturbed. Turn off the ringer on the phone. Close the door to the room
and the outside world for this very sacred time. Let your family and pets
know that this is *your* time to *relax*.

It is helpful and conducive to your continued, regular practice of relaxation to have a designated place where you practice. At this place, keep two
blankets, two pillows, an eye pillow or cloth, an audiocassette player, and
tapes. If you are not using an instructional tape, one of soft soothing music
can help to block out exterior sounds and draw you deep within.

Allow yourself to lie down on a well-padded surface, so that you don't
feel any pressure points or sore spots. Have the feet about shoulder width
apart and place a pillow under your knees, high enough so the lower back
and abdomen are flattened. A pillow or rolled towel supports your head
and neck. Have the arms away from the body and, if comfortable, the
palms facing up. If lying on your back is not comfortable, this resting pose

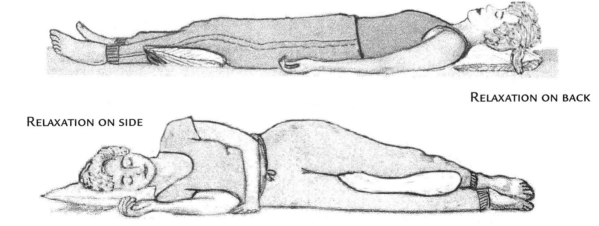

RELAXATION ON BACK

RELAXATION ON SIDE

can also be done while lying on either side with a pillow under the head and between the knees.

Place a soft cloth or eye pillow over your eyes to encourage them to relax. Made of silk and filled with flaxseed, eye pillows are wonderful accessories that aid in deepening the relaxation by keeping the eyes in total darkness and allowing them to be still. The stillness slows down the REM (rapid eye movements), which in turn slows the mind.

If you are sitting in a chair, allow yourself to be totally supported and the feet slightly elevated.

Cover yourself with a blanket, as the body temperature and blood pressure decrease with deep relaxation. You may feel chilled.

The blanket is also useful to evoke a nurturing and comforting feeling that allows you to feel safe and go deeper in relaxation. It may seem like the time we were in kindergarten, another good habit we lost along the way. Students always ask me, "Can we have milk and cookies when we get up from our rest period?"

"Yes, nonfat milk and nonfat cookies!"

Allow yourself this time to relax. All that needs to be done has been done. All you need to do now is let go and relax.

Since it is difficult to do deep relaxation while you read this, I suggest that you listen to the *Deep Relaxation* audiocassette from the Abundant Well-Being series or record your own voice reading the text and play it back for a deep relaxation. Using a cassette helps keep the mind focused and awake without the fear of falling asleep or missing an important appointment.

To fully experience the benefits of deep relaxation, allow the mind to stay awake as the body sinks into relaxation. For maximum benefit allow twenty to thirty minutes or longer of undisturbed practice time.

PRACTICE OF DEEP RELAXATION

Allow the eyes to close. Adjust the body so that it is comfortable and relaxed. Now you can totally let go.

Notice if there is more pressure on one side or another, if one side of the body is tighter or looser than the other, and remember to breathe evenly and gently and if possible through the nose.

STAGE ONE: *ANNA MAYA KOSHA*, PHYSICAL BODY

Bring the awareness to the right leg. Stretch out the right leg from the hips to the toes. Squeeze the right leg and be aware of all the muscles from the toes to the hip. Inhale; raise the leg a few inches. Exhale; relax the leg. Roll it gently from side to side and allow it to relax.

Bring the awareness to the left leg. Stretch out the left leg from the hips to the toes. Squeeze the left leg and be aware of all the muscles from the toes to the hip. Inhale; raise the leg a few inches. Exhale; relax the leg. Roll it gently from side to side and allow it to relax.

Bring the awareness to the right arm. Stretch out the right arm and splay the fingers. Make the hand into a fist. Squeeze the right hand and arm and be aware of all the muscles from the fingers to the shoulder. Inhale; raise the arm. Exhale; relax the arm. Roll it gently from side to side and allow it to relax.

Bring the awareness to the left arm. Stretch out the left arm and splay the fingers. Make the hand into a fist. Squeeze the left hand and arm and be aware of all the muscles from the fingers to the shoulder. Inhale; raise the arm. Exhale; relax the arm. Roll it gently from side to side and allow it to relax.

Bring the awareness to the buttocks. Inhale; gently squeeze the buttocks and feel all the muscles on both sides equally. Exhale; relax. Allow the buttocks to relax and soften as you feel the floor supporting them.

Bring the awareness to the abdomen. Inhale; expand the abdominal muscles. Exhale; relax and allow the abdomen to soften.

Bring the awareness to the chest and lungs. Inhale as the chest and lungs expand. Exhale; allow the chest, lungs, and heart to relax. Observe how the breath has become smooth and gentle.

Inhale; gently squeeze the shoulders up to the ears. Exhale. Relax.

Roll the shoulders back gently against the pillow or floor and away from the ears. Relax.

Observe the neck. Slowly and gently roll the head to the left and then to the right and back to center. Bring the chin down slightly toward the chest. Allow the head to find its natural center. Relax.

Bring the awareness to the face. Inhale; close the jaw. Exhale; allow it to open. Relax.

Observe the lips and cheeks. Inhale; squeeze them together. Exhale; relax.

Bring the awareness to the eyes. Inhale; squeeze them together. Exhale; relax. Observe them becoming soft.

Bring the awareness to the space between the eyebrows and the forehead. Inhale; raise the eyebrows. Exhale; relax. Feel an imaginary hand soothe away any tension on the forehead and all the worry lines. Allow your face to become soft and smooth.

Observe the heaviness of the physical body in its relaxed state as it is freed from the tightness of the muscles.

STAGE TWO: *PRANA MAYA KOSHA,* ENERGY BODY

Inhale deeply and on the exhalation, send the breath down the legs to the feet. Allow the feet to relax.

Inhale deeply and on the exhalation, send the breath to the ankles.

Inhale deeply and on the exhalation, send the breath to the calves and shins.

Inhale deeply and on the exhalation, send the breath to the knees.

Inhale deeply and on the exhalation, send the breath to the thighs and hips. Allow it to replace any tension or discomfort. Relax.

Allow the breath to return to normal.

Observe the feet and legs as they become heavy with relaxation.

Inhale deeply and on the exhalation, send the breath down the arms to the fingers. Allow all the muscles, nerves, and bones, etc., to relax.

Inhale deeply and on the exhalation, send the breath to the hands.

Inhale deeply and on the exhalation, send the breath to the wrists.

Inhale deeply and on the exhalation, send the breath to the forearms.

Inhale deeply and on the exhalation, send the breath to the elbows.

Inhale deeply and on the exhalation, send the breath to the upper arms and shoulders, allowing it to replace any tension or discomfort. Allow the breath to return to normal. Relax.

Observe the hands and arms as they become heavy with relaxation.

Notice how the limbs feel very heavy and still, how they weigh down the rest of the body like anchors. When the limbs are still and heavy, it encourages the rest of the body to be still.

Inhale deeply and on the exhalation, send the breath to the buttocks.

Inhale deeply and on the exhalation, send the breath to the pelvis and pelvic organs.

Inhale deeply and on the exhalation, send the breath to the abdomen and allow all of the abdominal organs to relax, releasing blocked energy from all the pelvic and abdominal organs.

Inhale deeply and on the exhalation, send the breath to the chest, lungs, and heart.

Inhale deeply and on the exhalation, send the breath to the throat. Allow the breath to return to normal. Relax.

Observe the front of the body as it becomes soft with relaxation.

Inhale deeply and on the exhalation, send the breath to the lower back and spine, to each vertebra, muscle, and nerve.

Inhale deeply and on the exhalation, send the breath to the midback and spine.

Inhale deeply and on the exhalation, send the breath to the upper back and spine, between the shoulder blades and the heart.

Inhale deeply and on the exhalation, send the breath to the shoulders, neck, and base of the head. Allow the breath to return to normal. Relax.

Observe the back as it comes closer to the floor in relaxation.

Inhale deeply and on the exhalation, send the breath to the entire brain.

Inhale deeply and on the exhalation, send the breath to the jaw, allowing it to replace any tension or discomfort. Relax.

Inhale deeply and on the exhalation, send the breath to the lips and tongue. Relax.

Inhale deeply and on the exhalation, send the breath to the cheeks and nose. Relax.

Inhale deeply and on the exhalation, send the breath to the eyes, behind the eyes, and eyelids. Allow the eyes to soften and relax.

Inhale deeply and on the exhalation, send the breath to the forehead and temples. Relax.

Inhale deeply and on the exhalation, send the breath to the sides of the head, temples, and the ears. Relax.

Inhale deeply and on the exhalation, send the breath to relax the scalp. Allow the breath to return to normal and allow the entire face to soften and become smooth like the face of a baby.

Observe the body. Notice if there is any part of the body that does not feel completely relaxed. Go back to that part, inhale, and as you exhale encourage it to relax.

Notice how the body has become very heavy with relaxation. Observe the heaviness of the legs, arms, back, head—knowing you are able to move, if necessary, at the same time not wanting to. Enjoy the feeling of letting go.

STAGE THREE: *MANO MAYA KOSHA,* BODY OF THE MIND AND SENSES

Observe the breath once again. Notice how still it becomes as the body relaxes. Observe the breath without controlling it as it comes and goes without any strain. It is so gentle you can barely feel the chest moving.

Guide this gentle breath to remove any subtle tension, thoughts, feelings, or memories in the feet; gently brush the ankles, lower legs, knees, thighs, hips. Relax.

Guide this gentle breath to remove any subtle tension, thoughts, feelings, or memories in the fingers, hands, wrists, forearms, elbows, or upper arms. Letting go of what you are holding with the hands and arms, send the gentle breath to the shoulders. Let go of your burdens. Relax.

With that gentle breath, touch the buttocks and pelvis, allow the abdomen to soften, touch the chest, lungs, and heart, releasing old pain and hurt; touch the throat, releasing any unsaid words. Relax.

Send the gentle breath to the base of the spine and allow the breath slowly to come up through the middle spine to the upper spine, releasing deep-seated heartache from behind the heart. Relax the shoulders and allow the neck to be an open connection between the heart and head. Relax.

Gently relax the jaw, cheeks, and nose. The eyes soften and draw into the inner sight. Relax the eyelids, forehead, and ears as they draw inward to the inner sounds. Relax the entire scalp and bathe the brain with relaxation.

Observe the last bit of tension leaving the body through the top of the head. Relax.

Allow the gentle breath to touch the mind and feel all the subtle thoughts. Relax.

STAGE FOUR: *VIJNANA MAYA KOSHA,* BODY OF HIGHER WISDOM

Slowly bring the awareness to observe the gentle breath as it enters and leaves the body.

As it enters, feel it bringing vital energy and healing energy.

As it leaves, feel yourself letting go of thoughts, feelings, tensions.

Notice a lightness and a feeling of detachment from the body, mind, and all worldly cares.

(Have one full minute of quiet time.)

STAGE FIVE: *ANANDA MAYA KOSHA,* BODY OF BLISS AND JOY

Begin to go further within your heart to look for that place of stillness, peace, and joy. This is *your* place of ultimate relaxation, a wellspring of healing energy. Find that place and rest there.

(Have five full minutes of quiet time.)

Slowly and gently bring the awareness back to the breath. As we slowly relaxed the body, we will now gradually awaken the body.

Begin to increase the inhalation and feel energy entering with the breath and awakening the body.

Observe the body recharging with fresh, vital energy.

As you inhale, feel the energy come through the top of the head.

Inhale; guide the energy down the spine to its base. Exhale.

Inhale; revitalize the internal organs. Exhale.

Inhale; embrace the heart with healing energy. Exhale.

Inhale; fill the lungs and feel the throat open. Exhale.

Inhale; allow the energy to move down the arms to the fingers. Exhale.

Inhale; allow the energy to move down the legs to the toes. Exhale.

Observe the body as it tingles with vital, healing energy.

Keeping the eyes closed, continue to inhale and exhale deeply as you slowly move the toes, fingers, legs, and arms. Gently roll the head from side to side. Stretch out the body.

Observe how deeply relaxed the body is in its awakened state.

Observe how deeply relaxed the body and mind have become.

Slowly allow the eyes to open halfway and observe that you are deep within, looking out through the windows of the soul. Notice how the world looks to you as the first ray of light enters your eyes.

Allow the feeling of peace and stillness that is your essential nature to spread through your life and share it with all you meet.

"HOW BEAUTIFUL IT IS TO DO NOTHING, AND THEN REST AFTERWARD."

—*Spanish proverb*

The Affirmation of Life—Breath

THE GREEKS CALL it *pneuma;* the Hebrews call it *ruach;* many call it the *gift of life.* Most simply call it *breath.* It is indeed the gift we are given as we take up residence on this earth—the affirmation of life.

As we begin our descent through the birth canal into the earth's environment, on some deep level we are aware that all will be different in a very short time. From the warm, dark, form-fitted sanctuary of our mother's womb we are thrust into the cold, bright openness of earth. We must at once take in this new atmosphere in order to survive. Almost simultaneously we announce our presence with a cry that affirms our new dependence on that substance called air.

We continue with the ritual of inhaling and exhaling for the rest of our lives. The amount we take in is regulated by our will to live—by our lungs, nervous system, posture, and especially our physical and emotional output. Approximately sixteen times a minute—day and night—each time we draw in the precious air we affirm our life on this planet. With each exhalation we let go. And whether the next breath will come in, none of us know.

We easily make plans for twelve, fourteen years from now. Yes, we may make plans, but no one knows for sure if they will happen. The only time we are sure of is right now. Here I am right now, in the moment. I'm happy to be here right at this moment. Life and breath go on in this moment. Realizing all this changes everything. It changes one's whole outlook on life.

One day we will breathe out and let go for the last time. Returning the air to its rightful owner, we leave the earth-made body. We as spirit leave. As we cried on our arrival and others cheered, now we go in peace and others cry.

In breathing, we are satiated—not just with oxygen but with vital energy. We inhale precious energy called *prana, chi, qi.* This is the same life force we extract from food, light, and love. The *prana* secures our body's health through the proper digestion of food, warding off diseases and fostering an overall sense of well-being. The clearer and stronger the life force essential to our survival is, the better we look and feel. When our minds become clear, decisions are easier; the emotions find their right place and bring us renewed fulfillment in even the smallest things we do. Life can sail along at a smoother pace without so many bumps and valleys when this energy is *balanced.*

This concept of energy may be somewhat unfamiliar to you. It is subtle, quiet, yet powerful and dynamic. It is an essential key for understanding who we are and why we get sick.

Although we take in *prana* in many ways, the breathing practices are the most effective way to channel that life force into all parts of the body and mind.

As you might remember from Chapter 3, Deep Rest, Deep Relaxation, the *Prana Maya Kosha,* or energy "body," is the second "body" or sheath. The breath is the bridge between the body and mind. It is the filling between the physical body and the mind-body sandwich. Its function is to act as the force of motion for the two other parts of the sandwich. Without energy the physical body cannot move. That is why when the energy leaves a body we consider it dead. When we are exhausted, we might say, "I am dead tired," meaning we are unable to access any energy to move the body.

Movements in our body affect our breathing. When we suddenly run or quicken our pace, the oxygen and energy requirements go up and we breathe faster. When we slow down, our breath follows.

The opposite is also true. As our breathing pattern changes our body is affected. If we are tired, a deep breath can fill us with vital energy, making us more alert.

The pattern of breath also directly affects the mind. It becomes a great aid for calming as well as energizing the mind. Sometimes we are "too tired to think." At other times the mind is "racing." For thoughts to move, they must have energy. Within the mind are millions of thought waves. They move about fast or slow, rhythmical or chaotic. The rhythm is in relationship to the breath and body movement. When we breathe slowly—especially on the exhalation—it gives our thoughts space to spread out. Because we're allowing space between the breaths, there is space between the thoughts. By spacing the thoughts, the pace is slowed, making the difference between something enjoyable instead of stressful. In music, spacing is very important. The more space between the notes, the more relaxing the music.

Awareness of the breath can bring vitality and enjoyment to each moment of life. By exhaling slowly, we know immediately if any strain or stress has crept into our body or mind. Our breath becomes a great barometer for relaxation *and* stress.

Wouldn't it feel great to be so comfortable and relaxed with a project or adventure that you could keep going as long as you wanted? The sustained energy floats the body and mind like a boat on the water rather than having to always push it along.

Regulating the breath can help in many situations during the day. When you find yourself agitated with daily irritants, notice your breath. Chances are you are taking in a breath, holding it, then letting it out quickly. Take a moment and adjust the pattern—in and out without hesitation or strain. If you are very upset, this will be difficult to do. If possible as soon as you notice yourself starting to become tense or the breath is irregular, take a few deep breaths and notice the thoughts and feelings calming down. Stay with it for a minute or longer and you will be amazed at how effectively it works.

When children witness a frightening event, as major or minor as it may seem to us, they come breathlessly running in to tell us about it.

The words and breath tell you the child is upset: *"Momommy! hahuha* (hic) *ahhh hahu* (sob) *waa!!!"*

"Sweetie, I can see you are very upset, but I can't understand what you're saying. Please calm down. What are you trying to tell me?"

Meanwhile, you have visions of a horrible incident that's just taken place. Your imagination is running wild. You are not getting any concrete information from him. You want to be able to calm him down but how? Taking him into your arms, you say, "Sweetie, take a deep breath. Now let it out slowly. Again. Good. Now can you tell me what happened?" The words are now able to be understood. The crisis was not as large as you had imagined it.

Did you notice your own breathing pattern change when you were fearful of what might have happened? What you were witnessing and experiencing was the child's mind expressing itself through his breathing pattern. His breath was mimicking exactly how his mind was thinking. When the mind is reeling, confused and frightened, the breath follows. The child was trying to tell you what happened, but he couldn't because his breath—which is needed for speaking—guided by the mind, was too disturbed.

As adults, we have learned to control our breath and speech. The traumas of childhood become the everyday occurrences of adulthood. We compensate by holding our breath, trying to stop the thoughts. However, our speech pattern would sound like a child's garbled words if holding and controlling our breath had not become a habit. The thoughts in the mind are still chaotic and upset but we have learned to keep the stress inside and from that, disease can manifest.

Taking a deep breath is like combing the energy around us. When we first awaken in the morning and go to the mirror, our hair may be sticking out in all directions. We all learned early in life to take a comb or brush and smooth it down, allowing the hairs to go more or less in the same direction. Then we feel satisfied and look and feel a little more in control (at least of our hair!). Breathing practices do the same thing with our energy field. We align and "comb" the energy; it becomes smoother, calmer, and more focused. The focused energy becomes like a magnet, attracting like polarities to us.

In a plain piece of metal, all the molecules are facing different directions in chaos. A magnet is a piece of metal in which all the molecules are perfectly aligned—the north poles facing one way and the south poles facing in the opposite direction. If you stroke the two pieces together in one direction only, the magnet will drag all the other molecules in the plain metal into alignment with itself, causing a second magnet to emerge.

When we do the breathing practices right before meditation or an important task, it encourages all the five bodies to form an alignment. This alignment results in the energy, mind, and wisdom being able to focus and act as one.

Consciously withdrawing and redirecting this *prana* the mind becomes focused and bright.

A smart and successful young lawyer was working at the Los Angeles County public defender's office. This is a stressful job even at the best of times. He invited me to visit and see how our justice department functions. After a less-than-inspiring tour of the jail and courthouse, we went to his office for a cup of herbal tea. While sipping the tea, I noticed that his wall was covered with awards and plaques, honoring him for outstanding service *and* courtesy. This represented quite an array of accomplishments for such a young man. He then pointed out that the awards were not only from the *public defender's* office but also from the opposition—the *district attorney's* office. How could that be? Why would the opposition give an award to the rival? On TV we see that even if they are the best of friends outside, in the courtroom they are adversaries.

He saw me looking at the awards with a puzzled look. "Do you want to know my method?" he asked with a gleam in his eyes.

"Yes, tell us!"

"Well," he began slowly, "I usually go into the courtroom a little bit earlier than everybody else. As the other lawyers come in, they immediately start to bicker with one another. The fighting starts before the court is in session. I sit quietly on one of the benches toward the back. As inconspicuously as possible, I do alternate nostril breathing. This helps me clear my energy and center my mind. When it is time to try the case, I am ready to deal with the facts and not the personalities of my fellow attorneys. I win most of the time." That's a perfect example of centered energy in action.

Changes in our thoughts and feelings affect our breathing pattern. When we're relaxed, we breathe more slowly and deeply. As stress and tension accelerate with the perils of normal life, our breath becomes more rapid and shallow.

Observe your breathing pattern as you walk into a business meeting, when being introduced to someone special, or driving on the freeway. Make sure your breath is even. I am always teased about taking in a deep inhalation as I enter a freeway ramp. I then exhale, sending my breath and energy in front of me. Then my car and I follow the energy.

Use the breath also for getting in touch with the mind. Trying to calm an agitated mind is difficult. The state of the mind reflects on the breath, changing its pattern. It also reflects on the body. By exhaling slowly, we initiate a parasympathetic nervous system reaction, your heart and blood pressure slow down, and the loop continues to slow down your mind. At that point, you say, "Now what was it I was so upset about? Oh, yes, I remember. Oh, well, it's not so important after all." If it doesn't work on the first try, it will work on the fifth or the hundredth time. Don't give up. Nobody ever conquered anything by giving up. You will slowly begin to gain control over your mind.

At times of stress many of us withdraw from our physical bodies and draw into our minds and emotional bodies. If the shallow breathing is left undetected, that in itself becomes a signal of stress. As the body and the nervous system react to the shallow breathing, more stress is produced. The cycle is self-perpetuating.

At such times many of us introduce outside substances to help us release stress and anxiety, pushing it deeper within our bodies and minds. Many of the substances we take to calm us down actually do more harm than good. Drinking alcohol may give us a sense of calmness but can actually suppress or exaggerate an emotional reaction. The problem with suppression is that it is like taking a stick of dynamite, lighting it, and putting it in a trash can with the lid on. At some point, it will blow up. This can be on the physical, mental, or emotional levels. It is much more difficult to put the pieces back together after a blowup than to fix the problem in the first place. The best way to stop the cycle is to calm and control the mind with conscious deep breaths.

I was coming in to wish a friend happy birthday and noticed he was hunched over his coffee table, fretting. On closer observation, I saw he was filling out his income tax return. On even closer examination, he was also doing alternate nostril breathing.

"What is it you are doing?" I asked.

"Trying to stay calm while filling out my tax return."

This is good in theory, but in practice this method was not giving him full concentration on the tax form or the breathing practices. It would bring better results for both projects to spend a few minutes on conscious breathing first and then work on the tax forms. The mind would be more focused and work could be done in half the time. As stress crept back in (tax forms usually have a recurrent stress rate), he could stop for a breathing break. This is one of the many uses of the breathing practices and not counted as a gift on your tax return!

When teaching yoga to cigarette smokers, deep breathing is one of the main practices I use to help them quit. Instead of reaching for a hot, toxic gulp of air, inhale a big gulp of fresh, oxygenated, energy-rich air. Most people take in a really deep breath when inhaling cigarettes. Notice how deep into the lungs the smoke goes by observing how long it takes for the smoke to come out of the nose. If we could only take that deep a breath *without* the smoke, how great that could make us feel! Some smokers will report that the deep inhalation and holding gives them time to think, assessing a situation. Some even claim that it aids digestion. All these benefits can be gotten from a few deep breaths without the harmful side effects.

Today we read all the studies on secondhand smoke, telling of the toxicity. Did you ever notice how shallow your breath is when you are near someone who smokes? Also, notice how shallowly you breathe in a recycled environment like an airplane. Your natural reaction for self-preservation will activate when the body is given a danger signal.

In normal *shallow* breathing we take in about one pint of air. Coming down the bronchial tubes, the midlung gets the largest saturation of fresh oxygen. Since there is a limited amount of air that has been inhaled, the lower and upper lobes are not served with the same richness of oxygen as the midlung. We then have only the same amount to breathe out—about a pint of air. The upper and lower lobes are again unable to free the oxygen-deprived air they have stored.

As we inhale *deeply,* the diaphragm, a large dome-shaped sheet of muscle that separates the chest and abdomen, descends into the abdominal cavity. It is attached to the spine, ribs, and sternum. The muscle moves downward, causing a partial vacuum in the chest cavity that allows a larger quantity of air to flow into the lungs than when the diaphragm does not move.

When the diaphragm goes back to its relaxed position in an arc under the lungs, it gently allows the air to exhale from the lungs. That is why we begin our practice with the belly or abdominal breath. The diaphragm is also connected to the pericardium, the sac that surrounds the heart. When we take in a deep breath, the heart is gently massaged. The heart, being a muscle, loves to be massaged just like we enjoy having our shoulders or back muscles massaged.

As babies, we belly breathe, developing our lower lungs first. Much of our early months is spent lying down. Our physical activity is minor compared to our rapid *inner* growth and development. There is a gentle, rhythmical in-and-out motion as the belly expands and contracts. This enables the lower part of the lung, which contains a higher concentration of alveoli (air sacs), to develop and receive much-needed oxygen. The next part to develop is the middle part of the chest and lungs. Then, as more of the activity is either sitting or standing, the upper lungs or apex develops.

As adults we tend to keep the belly still when we breathe. Sometimes, for the sake of fashion or even in the military, we are taught to keep the belly sucked in. The first stage of the three-part breath is designed to relax and enable the belly to reunite with its use in breathing.

In deep three-part breathing, we take in a greater quantity of oxygen that allows for more efficient distribution to the lower, mid, and upper (apex) lung. This gives us more available oxygen *and* more life force or *prana.* All told, deep breathing allows us to take in about seven times the amount of oxygen as in our normal breathing. When we take in that slow, deep breath, the lungs fully expand and the entire system is oxygenated. There is even a special response that triggers a physiological response to persuade the body to *relax* with each exhalation.

The Breath and the Nervous System

Perhaps you can remember a time when you felt danger. You may have been walking down a street in the darkness. Suddenly you heard quick footsteps behind you. In a decision to fight or run you inhaled and then held your breath. As the footsteps came nearer and then ran past, you audibly exhaled in a sigh, "Ahhhh!" It was only a jogger out for a late evening run. Your body and mind were getting ready for danger.

Take this scene and change it slightly to a car pulling out in front of you or a child chasing a ball into the flow of traffic or even running for a ringing phone.

Notice your breathing pattern after one of these events. The inhalation primarily relates to the sympathetic nervous system, which encourages us to take action or run. The exhalation relating to the parasympathetic nervous system assists us in letting go and returning to balance after the danger has passed: "Ahhh!" With the balance of inhalation and exhalation, we are able to stay centered and focused, reacting appropriately to each situation as it occurs.

Most of us in chronic stress are taxing our sympathetic nervous systems too much of the time. As these stressful situations become more and more a regular part of our lives, they affect us on a deep physical and emotional level. When we are in the habit of holding our breath or breathing shallowly, our health and emotional outlook on life is affected. Our bodies become deprived of the energy and nourishment they need to live fully. By breathing shallowly or irregularly sixteen times a minute, we are constantly reinforcing a negative affirmation for life.

While I was teaching in Italy, a colleague of mine asked me to visit her father. He had advanced stages of emphysema and was having trouble breathing; she hoped I could teach him to breathe more deeply. Since he was a very proud man, he was unable to take any counsel from his daughter.

With an overoptimistic attitude, I went to see him one bright sunny afternoon. His flat was dark and all the curtains were sealed shut. His welcome was less than warm as we sat down in the living room.

"Well," he sarcastically began, "I suppose you are here to tell me not to drink wine or eat meat."

"No," I said as sweetly as I could.

"Then what *are* you here for? To teach me to breathe?"

"Just to talk," I said, even sweeter than before.

"Talk? Talk about what?" he wheezed.

"Nothing in particular. Just to get to know each other." I sat still and quiet. I silently prayed to have some insight, to be able to be of some service to this suffering man.

We politely began to speak to each other. Somewhere in the back of my mind, I was remembering that in Chinese medicine the lungs are related to sadness and sorrow. I wondered what this fact had to do with this tough man in obvious physical distress. Knowing that Tony was American-born, I began our chat with the simple question "What brought you to Italy, and why did you stay and raise your family here?" I asked the question and then listened in stillness, with both ears and heart open.

The answer that followed amazed and kept me spellbound for the next two hours. It has stayed in my heart to this day. Tony, a major in the U.S. Army during World War II, had been in charge of the first troops to enter Italy. In more detail than I wanted to hear, he described what atrocities he encountered. I found myself becoming breathless as his words turned into irregular and muffled emotional drawings. Tears started to well and drop from his lower eyelids. I had to stop myself from getting up for a tissue, fearing the movement would distract or disturb the fragile tissue paper atmosphere. I felt it would dissolve if I moved even an inch. He continued unashamedly as he described his moves through the war-torn villages, finding orphaned newborns, some still alive.

After what seemed like a lifetime and a second all in one, the spell was broken. His tear-streaked face looked years younger than an hour ago. He looked at me with great vulnerability and said, "I never told this to anyone ever. I don't know why I revealed all this to you now." Both he and I felt very hesitant about the next move. I was more certain than he and got up for a tissue to wipe the streaked sorrow from his skin.

After my solemn promise not to tell his daughter or family, we broke the veil and moved into the other room—or what seemed like another realm. I felt that I had all this knowledge about this man in my cells. Open to learning, Tony wanted to strengthen his body and mind from the ordeal they had been reliving each day for the last forty years.

Observing his breathing pattern immediately substantiated his physical and emotional struggle. His breath was shallow and labored, and it became painfully obvious that he was a reverse or paradoxical breather. This was how his body, mind, and breath responded to processing unfathomable grief and untold and repeated fear. With great powers of concentration and a little help from me, he tried to correct this old habit of destructive breathing patterns.

Reverse breathing is a habit that is born out of being frightened over and over again. As we feel fear, our "normal" sympathetic response is to inhale and hold the breath. This allows the blood to be shunted to our extremities supplying the energy needed to fight or flee. With this inhalation, the belly is also sucked in—as if the wind has been knocked out of us. This is the opposite position the abdomen takes in a normal inhalation. We then hold the breath in until the danger passes. Quickly, with an outward and audible sigh, the breath and belly release.

In our normal, relaxed breath, the lungs are inflated as the belly expands. The diaphragm moves down into the abdomen to allow more extension of the lungs. In reverse breathing, the belly tightens, basically saying, "No room here." When we breathe this way we are actually fighting our body's own natural flow.

If this breathing pattern becomes chronic, the breathing is restricted and insufficient. Each time we inhale improperly, we unknowingly trigger a fear response in our bodies and minds.

In most cases this reverse breathing can *easily* be corrected by focusing on the correct way to breathe. (If you suspect that you may be reverse breathing, there is an explanation on how to correct reverse breathing later in this chapter.)

One of the interesting parts of this breathing process is that when one is asleep, the reverse breathing reverts back to normal breathing. Is that fear memory stored in the *body or mind?*

Tony practiced diligently and was able to correct his longtime reverse breathing pattern. I hope that through my stillness and compassion he was able to melt some frozen grief and begin to live with the fearlessness and hope that he administered to others some fifty years before.

As we begin to expand the chest and lungs in deep inhalations, we find the air flows in easily. The lungs relax and the air seems to leave the body by itself. The diaphragm then pushes gently against the lungs to coax out the last bit of air. As you develop control, you'll find that the exhalation is effortless.

Observe your breath and notice whether the inhalation or the exhalation is longer. Most of us inhale for a longer time than we exhale. This can also be interpreted as a statement about our society. We want to take in as much as possible and give out as little as possible.

With the continuation of the breathing practices, the exhalation will gradually increase until it becomes twice as long as the inhalation. We focus on the exhalation, the letting go. The inhalation then comes back in naturally. To get the feeling of a deep exhalation, verbally sigh on the slow exhalation: Ahhhhhh! We're not breathing out twice as much air, but we're taking *twice the time* to breathe out. By encouraging a long, slow exhalation, the parasympathetic nervous system is activated and toned, allowing us that feeling of relaxation.

Breathing this new, deeper way actually encourages the heart to rest. The heart, being a great servant, rests only in between beats. Long exhalations give the heart more time to relax.

These simple lessons from the heart and breath can change our view of living in this world. When we have time to rest and nourish ourselves, we then can enjoy giving twice as much as we receive.

Perfect Design

The nose is the perfect vehicle for breathing. Whoever designed the nose did a great job. It has two equal tubes that moisten and an intricate system of fine hairs that filter the air. If you or your ancestors are from a hot, dry climate, your nose may be long and thin. This design provides more area for the air to be filtered and moistened. If you are from a hot, moist climate, your nose will be shorter with large nostrils as the air needs less processing to be acceptable to the lungs. The cold regions produce noses that are long and wide, warming the air. The nose is so well designed for this work there's no need to encourage the mouth to be used for breathing.

The mouth is designed for large quantities of solids or liquids. It is however very handy as a stand-in if we have a head cold or when the nose is otherwise occupied or stuffed. It may seem curious to have two separate nostrils when most of the time we use them as one unit. Actually, the nose is lined with erectile tissue that causes the inside of the nose to swell *and* shrink. Although most of us are probably not aware of it, the lining of each nostril engorges and shrinks periodically during the day. This necessitates the flow of air to shift from one nostril to the other in a biological rhythm.

The right nostril, governed by the sympathetic nervous system, corresponds with the left side of the brain and the attributes of heat, thinking mind, intellect, and reason, sometimes thought of as masculine characteristics. The left nostril, governed by the parasympathetic nervous system, corresponds with the right side of the brain and the attributes of coolness, intuition, feelings, and knowing, sometimes thought of as feminine characteristics.

Extreme heat or cold can also *cause* the nostrils to change or switch dominance. A desired heating or cooling effect is produced by allowing the air to pass through either the right or left nostril respectively. If you are outside on a cold winter day—even though you are not aware of it—your right nostril is fully open and desperately trying to heat the body. When you suddenly change your environment and walk into an over-heated store, your right nostril will shut down and the left will go into action.

This switching pattern becomes more obvious when you have a head cold that stops up your nose. Usually one of the nostrils at a time opens enough to let some air flow through.

Mental states can also change the dominance. When we feel anger or passion, heating emotions, chances are our right nostril will be dominant. Depression or compassion may cause the left nostril to open. At night, as the nostril dominance shifts, we turn from one side to the other. Whichever side we are lying on, the opposite nostril is open. If you are taking a nap in the heat of day the right nostril is less dominant, allowing you to rest and even dream. If the phone rings suddenly and wakes you up from your sleep, the left nostril will engorge, allowing the right nostril to open so you are able to be present for the call. The body's consciousness is awake even when we are sleeping.

The ancient system of Yoga appreciates that the two nostrils function separately. The breathing techniques, especially alternate nostril, were developed to help "rebalance" the equilibrium of breath and the mind. When equanimity is reached, we feel balanced in body, mind, and spirit.

If the nostrils are not fully open, there are ways to open and clear out the nose, allowing the breath to easily flow. The nasal wash technique helps to keep the nostrils clear and functioning properly. It involves atomizing or sniffing a warm, mildly salty (like tears) solution of purified (not chlorinated) water into the nose one nostril at a time. Allow it to stay for a short time and then gently blow it out. The salt water softens, dissolves, and washes away mucus and strengthens the mucous membranes. This allows them to function properly, warding off viruses, bacteria, and allergens.

Natural food stores have small teapotlike vessels for use in the nasal wash or any drugstore will have a baby nasal syringe. It is interesting that we routinely clean out babies' noses but not adult ones.

PRACTICE OF BREATHING TECHNIQUES

THREE-PART BREATH

The first part of the three-part breath or belly breathing can be practiced while lying down in the relaxation position or sitting comfortably with the back erect. The most important aspects are that you are relaxed, the belly is soft, and the energy is flowing in the spine. Keep the breath steady and gentle without any strain. If at anytime you feel dizzy or light-headed, discontinue the practice and allow the breath to return to normal. Remember to breathe through your nose, which filters and warms the air.

STAGE ONE: Place your right hand so that the thumb rests at the navel and the fingers embrace the belly. This will help you to be aware of the movement of the abdomen as you breathe. Begin by exhaling completely through the nose. The belly and the right hand will move in. At the end of the exhalation, slightly contract the belly.

Begin the inhalation by expanding the belly and the right hand, allowing the lower lungs to fill. As you exhale, contract the belly. Inhale and expand the belly; exhale and contract the belly. Continue a few times until you feel comfortable with the practice.

You may notice that you feel calmer and more relaxed after just this simple practice.

As you become comfortable with the first part (belly breath) of the three-part breath, you can add the second part.

STAGE TWO: Place your right hand on your belly and your left hand on the side of your lower ribs. Exhaling completely through the nose, inhale and expand the belly. Continue to inhale, allowing the lower rib cage to expand. Then exhale, allowing the breath to flow out of the rib cage area and middle lungs; then pull in the abdomen. Inhale and expand the abdomen and the rib cage; exhale and contract the rib cage and the abdomen; inhale and expand the abdomen and the rib cage. Continue parts one and two of the three-part breath until you feel comfortable with this part.

STAGE ONE

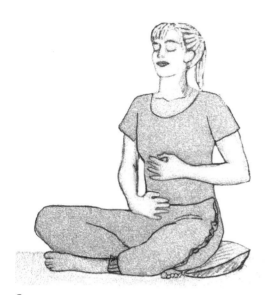

STAGE TWO

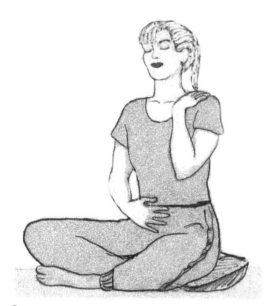

STAGE THREE

As you feel ready, end the breath with an exhalation and return the breath to normal. Relax.

STAGE THREE: For this next part, place your left hand on your upper chest. This is the third part of the three-part breath.

Exhale. Inhale and expand the belly and lower lungs, continuing to inhale to the upper chest. Feel the collarbones rise slightly. On the exhalation, release the air from the upper chest, the lower chest, and the abdomen—one section flowing into the other. Inhale and continue to expand the abdomen and lower chest, the middle chest and upper chest, so that the collarbones rise slightly.

Continue breathing slowly and deeply for a few minutes, ending with an exhalation.

By breathing this way, we are utilizing the full lung capacity, taking in approximately seven times the amount of oxygen in our normal shallow breathing.

The chest muscles and lungs may not be accustomed to such expansion, so be extra alert to any strain or dizziness. If you begin to get tired or short of breath, return to normal breathing for a few breaths, and then, after resting, continue the three-part breath. This will help build up your stamina without strain. Strain or stress actually depletes the life force, erasing many of the good effects from the breathing practice.

If you are comfortable with the breath and are in a prone position, experiment with sitting up with the spine erect and notice if it feels the same or is more difficult. Begin to adjust to doing the breathing practice in the sitting posture because you are upright much more frequently. Breathing this way will gradually become automatic if you practice it on a regular basis.

CORRECTING REVERSE BREATHING

If you do the three-part breath and notice that your belly goes in as you inhale and out as you exhale, you could be reverse breathing. Depending on how long you have been breathing this way, it may be easier or more difficult to correct.

Place both hands, fingers folded, across the belly and, as you exhale, press the belly in. Release with the inhalation. When lying down, you could use a book or a sandbag, anything with weight and pressure to aid the correct movement.

To get the feeling of the flow of breath, imagine there is some dust in your nose and you are trying to blow it out. Which way would your breath go? Out. Which way would your belly go? In. Doing that several times may often help correct the pattern. You may need to concentrate fully in order to correct a now automatic response. Don't get discouraged. You will really feel the difference in your energy and centeredness. The body wants to function as it is intended to; it will give you all the help it can.

ALTERNATE NOSTRIL BREATHING

As the pattern and flow of the breath becomes more natural, we can begin to regulate and balance the breath. Alternate nostril breathing is an exceptionally powerful technique for calming and relaxing your mind and body.

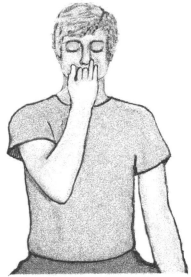

This breathing practice is done in a comfortable seated position. Use the same three-part deep breath as we did before. The only difference is that we are breathing through only one nostril at a time. The left hand is resting comfortably on the lap. With the right hand, make a gentle fist and release the thumb, the ring finger, and the little finger. This is a classical hand position of Yoga called Vishnu Mudra (seal). If it is uncomfortable, you can use the thumb and index finger. The thumb gently presses the right nostril closed while the left nostril remains open. Then the extended fingers gently close the left nostril and the thumb releases the right nostril.

To begin, exhale fully. Close off the right nostril with your thumb and inhale slowly through the left nostril.

Close off the left nostril with the fingers and exhale through the right nostril. Inhale through the right nostril. Close off the right nostril with the thumb and exhale through the left nostril. Continue this pattern. Exhale, inhale, switch nostrils; exhale, inhale, switch. Begin to practice for one minute and gradually increase up to three minutes or longer.

If at any time you feel any discomfort, simply resume normal breathing. As the breath becomes easeful, resume the alternate nostril breath. In this way you will gradually build up your endurance and stamina.

At the end of three minutes, as you come around to the right nostril, end with an exhalation. Allow the hand to come to the lap and be still with the eyes closed. Observe how calm and still the breath and mind have become. Observe the relationship between the two.

REGULATING THE COUNT

After you feel comfortable with the pattern of alternate nostril breathing, you can begin to regulate and bring balance to both nostrils.

Begin by counting how long it takes you to breathe in through the right nostril and how long to breathe out through the right nostril. Then do the same with the left, both in and out. They may be very different from each other. You may even have four different numbers. Begin to regulate the count of the inhalation, so that the lowest number from the inhalation is used. For example, if the inhalation count for the right nostril is three in and the left nostril inhalation is four in, adjust the count for both to three. Do the same with the exhalation.

Always use the lowest count and, as you relax, you may find the closed nostril opens. Then you can move the count on both sides up one count, in this case, to four.

It may vary each day. Begin each day anew. Instead of moving to where you were yesterday, be slow and gentle in expanding the count. Start with three and then move to four and maybe even to five. So what you are doing is instead of setting up a situation for failure and anxiety, you are setting it up for ease and to win. We want the challenge. Make it a win-win.

Continue to increase the inhalation and exhalation until they are equal to each other. When you are comfortable with a count of six in and six out, slowly begin to increase the length of the exhalation. From six-six move to six-seven, until the exhalation is twice as long as the inhalation. Savor the breath by letting it out more slowly. You are gaining more control and it takes longer to exhale completely. Just by equalizing the breath you are balancing the sympathetic and parasympathetic nervous systems. This allows you to feel the peace and calmness balance brings.

HUMMING BEE BREATH

This is a fun, yet very effective breathing technique for concentration and meditation. This breath helps to tone and balance the pituitary gland, which is located directly in the center of the head.

The pituitary gland looks like a pea on a stem that dangles down in a protective saddle filled with blood. As we know, sound moves quickly and is magnified by liquid. These humming sounds vibrate the blood and that in turn vibrates the pituitary gland. This results in a toning effect on the pituitary gland and, most of all, a real feeling of well-being. Try it before meditation or anytime you would like to have this feeling.

Sitting with the spine erect, take in a deep three-part breath. On the slow exhalation, keeping the mouth closed, make a humming sound within the head—feel it on or behind the soft palate. When the sound is gone, inhale and repeat the sequence. Repeat five times with different pitches—low, high, medium. Observe which sound vibrates where. Sit very still and enjoy the sense that everything is all right.

"IT IS NOT THE YEARS IN YOUR LIFE BUT THE LIFE IN YOUR YEARS THAT COUNTS."

—*Adlai Stevenson*

In breathing practices, we're enhancing the efficiency of our own breath while synchronizing the body, mind, and breath. One of the great things about meditation and breathing is that the goal is in the action of being still. Even if we get to the highest stage of the breathing practices, we're still sitting there with our breath.

The more these practices are used, the more they will show you the peace that is your own true nature. Enjoy.

CHAPTER 5

Dynamic Stillness—Meditation

"LIFE IS ALL

MEMORY, EXCEPT

FOR THE ONE

PRESENT

MOMENT THAT

GOES BY YOU SO

QUICKLY YOU

HARDLY CATCH IT

GOING."

—*Tennessee Williams*

ALBERT EINSTEIN, one of the greatest scientists of all time, was asked how he discovered the atom. "The atom," he said, "was not discovered. I meditated on it and it revealed itself to me."

Yoga, meaning "yoke" or "union," is described in the *Yoga Sutras of Patanjali* as transcending or gaining mastery over the thought waves of the mind. When the mind is in a state of Yoga, it is like a deep mountain lake, clear, still, and calm. We are able to see our true self reflected in it. We then know who we really are. At all other times we are constantly tossed around by the thoughts that come and go in the mind, clouding our view of who we are.

To achieve this state of peace and stillness, we practice steadying the mind. The Yoga sutras define three distinct phases to meditation. *Dharana* is *concentration,* or the beginning effort of steadying the mind on one point. Here the mind stays on the object of concentration for a few moments and then begins to run here and there in its usual pattern. *Dhyana* is *meditation,* which is the continuous flow of concentration, one-pointed focus. With meditation the mind focuses on the object for a longer period of time without fluctuation. *Samadhi* is *absorption,* when the mind and the object become one. Degrees of peace are obtained with each stage, waning with the demands of daily life. Only in the final phase, *Samadhi,* are our thoughts and mind steadied forever. One part of us always remains with our true self. The Bhagavad-Gita says, "The hand is in society and the heart is with God."

With all of our energy focused on one thought, all the other thousands of thought waves become impotent. We are able to move through the mind and experience our center, a completeness. Our true nature shines through.

When we delve into the practice of meditation, a yearning for peace and stillness blossoms. The seed, planted long before and hidden deep within, now takes a significant place in our everyday life. Some event has brought it to fruition. It could have been a narrowly escaped accident, an illness, the death of a loved one, a time alone with nature, something that called us from within. Those calls link us with our spiritual selves. We then need to take the time to nurture and water that seed. With zestful and dedicated care, the seed grows and allows us to see the world at many new levels, heights, depths.

As small babies, our minds were still and clear. It always amuses me to see a group of adults standing around quietly with smiles on their faces watching an infant sleep. Why do we enjoy watching a baby? We experience a sense of peace and stillness reflecting from the baby's mind. While watching the baby, our minds *remember* that *we* once felt that way.

From their stillness of mind, the babies' perspective on the world is quite different from ours. They are fed, changed, and cuddled. Most of the time all they have to do is whimper or cry and their simple needs are instantly met. Their view of people is so different than ours *because* of their small size and helpless state and calm mind. Wouldn't we see the world differently if most of the people we came in contact with smiled at us and said sweet words? We can say almost anything to babies and they'll smile at us—even if we say things that aren't so nice: "Oh, you look so silly without any hair!" It is the *way* we say it; our smile, vibration is what they react to, rather than understanding our words. If we said those same words to an adult, he might be our enemy forever. Babies' minds have not yet collected all the different thoughts, fears, and prejudices. Their lake is still clear. They radiate happiness and contentment, and we enjoy being around them.

Every time a thought wave enters the mind it is like a pebble being thrown into the lake. It makes a small ring or ripple. When the same thought or pebble is repeated over and over, it begins to shift the sand or the earth at the bottom of the lake toward the shore. As the sand accumulates in one place a *barge* is formed. Anytime a thought wave comes— even if the intention is for it to be a separate independent thought—the sand barge pulls it toward the flow of that one main thought. As that one thought gets stronger it becomes a tendency, a trait, and eventually our personalities.

As babies, we have few preferences and thought waves; we are contented. We get older and our choices and distinctions multiply: Girls wear pink; boys wear blue. We develop likes and dislikes: Girls like dolls; boys like trucks. You are a good girl if you wear dresses and play with dolls; you are not a good girl if you play with trucks. Our minds and thoughts become polarized, prejudiced. Confusion sets in, and our peace and contentment slowly start to evaporate. We begin to conform *or* rebel, either taking its toll on our quiet minds.

I was talking with a friend about the thought waves in her mind, explaining that all these little waves do not allow a clear reflection so whatever we see becomes distorted. She chuckled and said, "Come with me." We drove to the ocean. The sea was stormy. She pointed and said, "That is my mind—not a lake with ripples, but an ocean in storm. I feel like I have no control over my mind or my life." Trying to transcend or master the thoughts in the mind is, for many of us, more like trying to control the waves of an ocean in storm rather than a lake. It's the *nature* of thoughts in the mind to move and toss about.

Don't allow your meditation practice to become a struggle with your mind. Make the mind a friend, not an enemy. Remember, you and your mind are on the *same side*—the side of wanting to be calm and peaceful. If the mind becomes your enemy, you will never have peace; it will always find a way to agitate you. As a friend, it will find ways to help you find peace. Instead of *fighting* to control the thoughts in the mind, rise above them as if in an airplane. Get distance from them and look down and see how small and undifferentiated everything looks. Or, if you wish, dive down deep. Like a scuba diver, go below the waves and turbulence to the silence, calmness, and beauty. When our minds become still, we have a clear reflection of what is around us. Go deep within.

Meditation, while much more than a stress management technique, can be used to relieve and moderate stress. But to use meditation for *only* that purpose is like using a high-powered laser beam to cut bread. Meditation is a tool for *total transformation*. It opens us up to that all-pervasive feeling of peace, which we may experience as a dynamic stillness.

When practicing meditation for stress management, it's very difficult to gauge yourself or to even measure your *progress* in meditation. The benefits come from the inside and affect the outside. There are subtle benefits for a subtle practice. It's not like a lowfat diet where you can measure cholesterol changes or exercise where your muscle strength allows you to lift fifty pounds. One of the obvious benefits we *can* observe is that our mental "fuses" get longer.

Notice how you react to something that would *normally* have made you angry. Anger is a very powerful thought wave. This thought may pop up in the mind many times during a day. At first, you may be the observer of this angry thought: I *feel like* I am beginning to get angry. You are in the position of watching the anger. Not yet involved, you are still in control and able to change the thought and direction of the energy. After this angry thought is dropped into the lake, ten, twenty, or more times in one day the observation distance and time may get shorter: I *am* getting angry. You are still watching yourself moving toward anger. After thirty to forty times, the angry thought comes and you move so close to it that it appears you and anger are one. We can take out the "am." *I am angry* becomes *I = anger.* Many of the thought waves that come into the mind were borderline angry thoughts; they got swept up into the overpowering angry wave. It then becomes harder and harder to control the "almost" angry thoughts.

Observing and slowing the thoughts gives us a moment to watch the mind, to observe. This helps us lengthen the mental fuse and be in control and act appropriately even in disturbing situations.

Facing a situation that would have upset them previously, people have told me, "Maybe the meditation is doing something after all." They begin to see it with a calmer mind: It's not worth getting myself all upset over this. I'm sure there's a way to handle this without getting angry. Sometimes you may need to get angry at a particular situation.

This introspection allows you to go beyond the mind and senses and see the *perfection in every act* and act accordingly. These are the kind of "results" to look for.

When we are told a story or given a problem to solve, our minds need to be open and clear. Otherwise it is *colored* by our thoughts. When we are looking at the world through rose-colored glasses, everything looks rosy, or when we see through a black cloud, everything looks dark. Use your discriminating mind to help you make decisions from a better perspective.

It always amazes me to listen to the way a small group of people report the witnessing of a traffic accident. Each person represents the prominent thought wave in *their* mind, casting an opinion or point of view. Sometimes they agree on what they have witnessed; more often they do not. Each mixes in his or her own opinion, experiences, thoughts, and emotions. Sometimes each comes up with an entirely different story.

Doing my civic duty, I was selected for a jury trial. Since I had an unusual name at the time (Swami Nischalananda) and was wearing long orange robes, I was surprised to be chosen to actually sit on a jury. The defendant was charged with evading a police officer. There was very little direct evidence and the trial lasted only two hours. At that time, the jury was directed to meet and decide if the defendant was guilty or not guilty. As we gathered in a separate room, it was fascinating how many stories and prejudices appeared. We had all seen *Perry Mason, Matlock, L.A. Law,* and other television dramas about attorneys; some of the jury members *played* prosecutor and some defender. One woman said she was sure the defendant was innocent because the policewoman could not be trusted. When we asked why, she said, "She carried a gun on her hip and that's inappropriate for a woman." One man was sure the defendant was guilty because all people who ride motorcycles are running from the police. It was a wonderful exhibition of how the conclusions were influenced by the thought waves of the mind. The debates continued. It was now close to dinnertime and starting to snow. I was firmly convinced that he was innocent and was not in any rush to go home. The other jurors were more anxious to leave. One by one as the clock ticked on, my fellow jurors moved over to my way of thinking. Finally, the verdict of not guilty was presented.

Curious, I asked the defense lawyer why he *chose me* for the jury out of all the other possible "normal" people. "I felt you had an open and honest heart, and would be fair."

Meditation is an unusual and somewhat difficult practice for many people, especially in the West. In our culture, our society, we are not rewarded or even encouraged to be still. I don't know how many of you—when you were children—were told to stop daydreaming and pay attention. I was one of those children who had notes sent home from school each report period: "She is a very intelligent student but does not apply herself. She spends her time daydreaming." Can you relate to that? Children seem to do that naturally. It is a way of taking a mini vacation from the place or situation that causes you stress. Our society discourages that, calling it *a waste of time.*

Many of us consider our quiet time the hours we spend reading newspapers, magazines, and books, watching TV, or listening to music. Our bodies may be still—even calmer than usual—yet our minds may remain very active.

As adults, when we begin to learn to be still and quiet, it is a difficult and sometimes tedious process. At times it seems to be an unnatural process. I want to acknowledge this because it is important not to get discouraged with meditation. Cultivating new habits takes time. Speak to a great singer or pianist. How many years did they practice to become great? How much time did they struggle with their minds? They probably wanted to do other things instead of practice. Even after they become accomplished, each day they go back to the beginning and practice the scales.

We sometimes feel, "Oh, I've been doing meditation now for two weeks and I've felt nothing." Even after practicing meditation for twenty and thirty years, the main benefits reside on the subtle, not necessarily on the physical levels.

As is often the case with meditation, we think everyone else is easily able to focus and go deep within and that we are the exceptions. In actuality we are all very much alike, with our minds running here, there, and everywhere. The mind has been described as a monkey—actually a drunken monkey and not just a drunken monkey, but a drunken monkey stung by a scorpion. The mind tends to dart in many different directions, everywhere except where we want it to be—focused on the meditation technique.

Sometimes, even when we hear it from an expert, our minds are in doubt. His Holiness the Dalai Lama was holding a retreat for a large group of people. Each day he would lecture on the different aspects of meditation and its presence in daily life. Patiently he would explain that the only way to feel the benefits was to practice, practice, practice. It may take years to experience a sense of peace that permeates our everyday lives.

Each day, before and after his talks, there was a period of meditation. Again in the evening, he would patiently and compassionately answer questions.

One man who had been at the retreat all week raised his hand and asked, "All this takes so long. Isn't there an easier and quicker way to get to this place of peace?"

The Dalai Lama cradled his head in his hands. He remained that way for about five minutes. When he finally raised his head, his face was streaked with tears. His eyes lit upon the many faces in the audience, as if to absorb understanding.

After what seemed like a long time, he began to speak slowly. With his hands balled up into fists, he chanted, "THERE IS NO EASY, QUICK WAY! THERE IS NO EASY, QUICK WAY! THERE IS NO EASY, QUICK WAY!"

Don't give up or get disillusioned with meditation. If you need results, look for long-term results, not quick ones. All great accomplishments take time. By daily, vigilant practice, the benefits will transform your body, mind, and spirit.

As medical science studies the effects of meditation on the body we begin to understand why many of the ancient sages lived a long, healthy life. In meditation, the body and the mind become relaxed and efficient, which produces the effect of lowering blood pressure, increasing immune function, and allowing us to feel vital with a greater sense of being in control of our lives. In The Lifestyle Heart Trials, we found that those who did the most Yoga practice, including meditation, each day have seen the most benefit in reversing their coronary artery disease. Another study showed that people who did meditation after their first heart attack were significantly less likely to have a second one. The mind affects the body.

Perhaps what we're missing in our society is this time of going within and because we ignore that we're developing many stress-related diseases. Could these diseases be the modern way of drawing us away from the "busyness" of life so we can take the time to be with ourselves again, to "be comfortable in our own skins" as the French say, and to heal?

Peg was a nurse and was certain her prognosis was leading her to a swan song. Her fear of her family history of breast cancer led her to the drastic act of removing both of her normal breasts. "This is not uncommon," she tried to convince me, "when your mother, sister, aunts, and grandmothers all died of breast cancer. I had it done for my peace of mind."

As it turned out, her mind was so focused on cancer that even after her breast surgery she developed ovarian cancer. Before it could be diagnosed, it had metastasized to her liver and lungs. Some part of her accepted this as her fate, while another part wished she could extend her short life.

Her spiritual life became her focus and fervently created a structure for her inner life to emerge. She came to spend time with me because to her *intuitive* self it felt right.

"I know that soon the cancer will take over my whole body and I will die. I am still a physically young woman. I had hoped to see my children grow up. That hope is now gone. I also know that a large part of who I am will live on. Will you help me get more in touch with that spirit within?"

After a few initial sessions in meditation instruction, Peg could be seen sitting in the field or on her bed till all hours of the morning, meditating. It was clear by the feeling surrounding her that she was touching deep places of comfort and healing.

One early morning she gave a perfunctory knock on my door and without waiting for an affirmative answer, she burst into my room. Sitting on my bed, she was wide-eyed and wild. "What is it? What happened?" my voice croaked from sleep as much as surprise.

"I just retrieved an experience from somewhere deep in me that I had forgotten or buried, so horrific that every part of my body, mind, and soul are shaken." I sat up and braced myself for the energy and words of the event.

Her boyfriend was going to visit some friends in a city two thousand miles away. He had left early one morning while she was still in bed, half asleep. With a promise to call that night, he planted a kiss on her lips and was off.

Late that night a phone call came. It was not as she had expected.

About seven that night, she fell into a swoon. All the physical world suddenly became translucent; she was seeing through the veils. Feeling a sense of unease, she could "see" her beloved sitting in a strange place. Suddenly there was a gun pointing at him, with first one, then another explosion. He was gripping his belly and his pain was *their* pain. She felt it as a hot iron, bursting inside her belly, ripping at her insides. Fear, panic, and horror kept her paralyzed until the ringing of the phone wrenched her back to a solid physical form. The voice at the other end said that her boyfriend had been shot and killed by two bullets in the abdomen. She replaced the phone and closed a heavy curtain to the pain and memory of that horrid scene.

Peg had trusted the curtain to keep the pain from her and she had not remembered anything about that night for five years. Now, as she delved into the recesses of her soul, she found a monster that was unknowingly gnawing away at her day and night. This realization was like discovering a new part of her that she had forgotten existed. She was meeting a long lost friend who had suffered much—the fear, the crying, the awe of it.

The physical and emotional integration of this event was both difficult and easy at the same time. Slowly owning the experience as an important part of her emotional and spiritual life, Peg continued to practice meditation. She was getting to know *all* of herself, perhaps for the first time in many years.

A few months later I received a phone call.

"Have you heard about Peg?"

"No," I said preparing for the worst.

"Well, she went to see her doctor and she is completely free of any cancer. It is gone. She has had a complete, unexplained, spontaneous remission from her disease!"

What *actually* healed Peg we may never know. It is one of those situations we hesitate to call a miracle because we want God or the higher power to remain *anonymous.*

I later found out that there are more than fifty thousand such *unexplained* spontaneous remissions each year in the United States that are *reported.* We don't know how many happen to people who just never tell anyone. A doctor may tell her patient to go home and make arrangements to die. Two years later she sees them in the supermarket buying zucchini! The curious part is that no one in the *medical* community can explain it.

Most of us in "normal" everyday life flop around like we are on the rim of a wheel; sometimes we're up high and happy, then we start to come down, and pretty soon we're underneath the wheel and something is crushing us. Slowly we come out from under the crush and around and up again. Depending on one's life and power of rejuvenation, the cycles can be shorter or longer. In meditation, we start to move in, in, in, to the center, the hub of the wheel, where there is always steadiness. So, no matter what happens, it happens around us—it doesn't affect us as directly. We sit still and steady, observing the situations and dramas that occur. We participate in them, yet there's always a *distance*. There is always a knowing that whatever happens, we are in the center, observing.

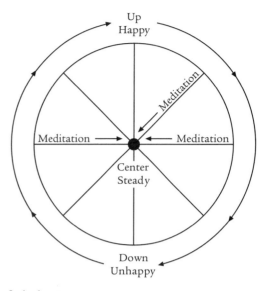

There was once a great and mighty king who had all the riches in the world. Nothing was beyond him in the physical sense, yet the king was unhappy. He realized that he could be happy for a short time by acquiring land, jewels, food, or drink, but his happiness always faded. He summoned all the healers, priests, and even jesters to help make him happy. Many people came to offer their suggestions, tricks, and charms. Nothing seemed to bring him the permanent happiness he wanted.

After weeks of exhausting interviews, a small, humble woman appeared before the king. "What could you possibly offer me that all the other great men and women could not?" he asked. The woman held out a velvet box. The king looked at the box and laughed. "You offer this great king jewels? I have the most precious jewels in the world."

"Excuse me, Your Majesty, but this is by far the most precious jewel. This can lighten all your sorrows and bring happiness into a troubled time."

The king's curiosity was piqued, so he took the box. Slowly he opened it and found a plain gold ring. "A plain gold ring!" he yelled and started to throw it away."

"Please, Your Majesty, read the inscription. Read it now and each time you are feeling happy or sad."

The king read the inscription and read it again as he relaxed on his throne: AND THIS TOO SHALL PASS.

Good, bad, happy, sad—all will pass. I actually had a stained glass with the inscription THIS TOO SHALL PASS given to me by one of my clients. I hung it over the desk in my office as a constant reminder.

By practicing meditation, we achieve a distancing from the outside of the wheel. It takes us literally into our center, into our spirit, into our self, into who we are. That's the purpose of meditation, to remind us to go back to our origin.

Meditation is not something that we *do*. We use techniques to get us to the point of meditation or stillness. Once we get to that point we are no longer *doing*, we just *are*.

Beginning the practice, we often expect to be able to just stop or immediately control our thoughts. In frustration, we say, "I can't stop my thoughts." Thoughts that have run wild for our whole life now, with one or two sessions, we expect to obediently come under control.

In meditation thoughts go by. They're not that important. Most of what we think about never happens anyway. Of all the plans we make, half of them never happen. Of all the worrying we do, most of that never happens either. Why waste that time? We experience frustration and a feeling that we are the only ones in the world unable to control their thoughts. So pull back from life's trials, watch them, and if you like, laugh at them.

Begin to observe the mind and thoughts as a movie screen. When one walks into a dark movie theater, there is only a plain white screen. Then suddenly something is projected on it and we get caught in the movie. Just as the scenes in a movie change, so do our thoughts and emotions in the mind. In the end, we realize that *life* is like a movie, just a *projection* from our mind.

There was once a great spiritual teacher who wanted to prove this very point to his students. He took a group of them to see a very scary movie. The teacher took his place in the row behind the students so he could observe them. "Now remember," he said, "this is just a movie."

"Oh, yes, we know," they repeated, "this is just a movie."

As the movie progressed and the frightening scenes came, the teacher observed the students leaning forward in their seats, tensing their bodies, some with pained looks on their faces. The teacher would then let out a roar of laughter. "Ha, ha, ha. You forgot. It is just a movie." Then they would remember and relax back in their chairs. Again, a few minutes later, they would forget and become tense again, and on and on it went. At the end of the movie, the screen went blank and the lights went on. It *was* a movie after all!

Our main objective in life is to remember—remember who we are in the midst of all the "busyness" of the outer world *and* our inner worlds.

Withdrawing our thoughts, feelings, and senses from the outside is *pratyahara,* which we learned about in the chapter on deep relaxation. In the beginning of practice, we identify the senses as they reach outward. We notice we are distracted by a truck passing by, someone turning a light on, or the temperature changing. Often we try to let the background noises be there without taking them in.

All of our senses have two components. As we draw further inward, we recognize the inner component of these senses. For example, our sense of hearing reaches out and reaches in. If you put your fingers in your ears right now, you would eliminate outer sounds and you might hear your heart beating. If you gaze at a candle with your eyes open and then close your eyes, you see the candle flame manifested with the inner eye. Have you ever had a flashbulb go off in your eyes when a picture was taken of you? You walk around for a few minutes with red and yellow dots in front of your eyes. You see the dots with the eyes open or with the eyes closed, the outer and inner sight.

Begin by withdrawing the senses from the outer world. The more we draw the senses inward, the less we are distracted by externals. And the less we are distracted by externals, the quieter the mind gets.

We then are conscious of our *inner* noises, thoughts shuttling back and forth in the mind. As we become still, we realize how much noise is created by the movement of our own mind. By our continually drawing in the senses, even the internal noises are quelled.

Many of us *choose* to be surrounded with background sounds. We have the television, radio, or stereo on all the time. It seems that we are trying to drown out the mind's noise by having louder noise outside—noise that we *can* control. It is difficult to truly experience outer quiet in our modern society. Just take a moment now and notice if your home is quiet. Is the refrigerator humming? Is a neighbor playing music or starting a car? Even the soothing sound of a bird is outside noise. We must go inside to experience real quiet.

A few years ago, I had the privilege of teaching some seminars in Australia. The retreat facility was far away from any town and was quite primitive by our standards. There were no television waves or even radio waves. When I arrived, after thirty hours in the whirl and whiz of a jet plane, I stood still, drinking in the absolute quiet that we rarely experience these days. Just being in the quiet led my mind to a state of calmness. It was an instant vacation.

Did you ever notice that even in very poor countries the places of worship are very beautiful? There we find the most beautiful artwork, the most sublime music, a literal feast for the senses. Why do you think that is? It is a very clever way of getting people to come and support the activity and the church. We may not be able to afford beautiful stained glass windows in our home or go to a great concert, yet we can appreciate them anytime by coming to a church or temple. Even if we can't pray, our senses are happily engaged looking at the beautiful windows, listening to the beautiful music. When the outer senses are soothed and satisfied we can more easily draw inward.

While sitting quietly in one of my favorite churches, Notre Dame de Paris, I noticed the tourists coming in to see the structure and the magnificent stained glass windows. I chuckled to myself as they were forced to *sit in the pews* to properly view the windows. Some of them, in spite of themselves, sat for a longer time, enjoying not just the windows but the sublime vibration that is palpably felt there. They came for one purpose, yet their higher nature seized the opportunity to be nourished.

The more senses we can engage, the stronger the experience is. We can see that today with the multimedia experience. No longer do we just go in and *see* a simple movie, we must also hear it from speakers that surround us. In one theater I actually experienced rain falling on me! Of the many senses we are able to engage on the outside, let them then draw us inward to greater focus on our meditation.

Whenever we are choosing tools for our work or play, we must take the time to select the correct size, shape, texture, and level of use. I may like the look and feel of advanced skis, yet if I am a beginner, the skis designed for beginners suit me best. When selecting food for a special meal, we prefer food that is tasty as well as nutritious. It is with that same consciousness that we embrace a meditation technique. Today there are many great techniques to choose from. The goal of any technique is to keep the mind engaged and focused until it becomes still.

The *Yoga Sutras of Patanjali* is very empowering and nonrestrictive. It simply suggests two criteria for selecting an object of concentration or meditation.

The first criterion is that it allows you to be both uplifted and inspired by just thinking about it. From there you can choose almost anything you wish. It can be a place or part of nature—perhaps remembering a time you stood transfixed looking at a sunset, so taken by its beauty, or sitting in front of a roaring fire, captured by its warmth and radiance, or it could be remembering a great soul you admire. Let it be something whose qualities, when you meditate on it long enough, enhance your character and well-being.

The second criterion is that you love it. Select something that makes you feel happy. When you pick a meditation technique that you love, the result is that you use it more and focus on it with greater concentration.

Many of us have had the experience of falling in love. When that first happens, our whole world and attention is geared to that one person—all of our senses, our thoughts are with them and just thinking about them uplifts us and makes us happy. *What will he want to eat? This is her favorite flower.* Imagine you're at an airport waiting for that special person you love so much. As you're standing there, waiting for the aircraft to come in, your feet may hurt a little bit, but the moment you see your sweetheart, it's as if all the energy comes out of your feet, moves up through your body, and leaps out through your heart.

Most of us have had that experience at some time in our lives. The experience of meditation may not be so dramatic. Yet, with time and practice, the centers of higher consciousness in our hearts and minds open and allow us to feel and know the higher truths.

Adopt a technique familiar and comfortable to you, something you can embrace as you would a close friend.

A friend of mine who has a longtime career as a cardiac surgeon went on a ten-day meditation retreat. When he returned, I casually asked him how the experience had been for him. "Oh, it was fine," he answered, still somewhat preoccupied. "Tell me something," he said. "They told us to meditate on the *hara* [an energy center used in Buddhist meditation]. I spent the whole time trying to figure out exactly where it was. Using my memory, I went through my copy of *Gray's Anatomy*, but I couldn't figure out if it is to the left or right of the pancreas, above or below it. Can you help clarify it for me?"

Half chuckling to myself and at the same time appreciating his dilemma, I said, "Let's make this easy. Do you know where your heart is?"

"Of course I know where my heart is—and everybody else's, too," answered the experienced surgeon.

"Put your full and complete attention at the heart, with all the love that flows through it. That is a grand object for meditation," I said. He looked relieved and a slight smile appeared in his sparkling eyes.

When you actually select a technique, feel a certain one-pointed devotion. Sometimes, in our impatience, we feel, *Oh, this technique is not working.* We speak to a friend or read a book about a certain method and decide to change our technique. We need to give our chosen technique time to go deep. There's an adage about digging shallow wells: If you dig down ten feet in one well and hit rock and ten feet in the next and you still are not getting water, you can keep digging many ten-foot wells and never reach water. But if you dig only one well and just dig thirty or forty feet deep straight down, you will eventually get water.

By switching techniques back and forth, you're not getting the depth and steadiness that you need. It is like buying a fire extinguisher and each week moving it to a different place. When the fire comes, you will not remember where to look. Becoming familiar with your technique allows you to go more quickly to the quiet and stillness within.

Just embrace one technique you feel is the closest to your temperament. Date it for a while. You don't have to get married to it, but at least keep steady company with it. Then, if you decide in three or four weeks that it is not for you, select another technique. Stay with that one for a month or so. After two or three tries, make your marriage plans and choose one. Apply that devotion to your technique and go deep within.

There is a certain benefit to keeping the technique sacred and not speaking about it to others. Much has been said about this and many people laugh at it. Yet our cherishing and valuing an object makes it sacred. If I were to pull a gold and emerald ring out of a popcorn box, you might doubt it was real. However, if I invited you into my room and closed the door, then unlocked a drawer and took out a velvet box, you would anticipate an expensive jewel. Much of our regard comes from our intention. If we feel we have chosen a special and very powerful meditation technique, it will be so.

Distractions in Meditation

We all have busy lives—filled with lists, time commitments, and too little time to do them. When we're sitting for meditation, all of these thoughts come rushing to the front of our minds. There are three main ways to get rid of obstacles (thoughts that come into our mind and demand our attention).

Sometimes it is easier to observe how our adult minds work by observing small children. They have not yet learned to cloak their ways as adults have. In the quiet of meditation, our minds tend to lose their cloaking device and become as transparent as when we were children. See if you can relate the obstacles that occur during meditation to this observation of small children.

Talking with a friend, her children felt ignored, left out. They interrupted the conversation, "Excuse me, Mommy. Mommy, Mommy, excuse me, Mommmmmy." The first thing she did was try to ignore the interruption. That is also the first thing to do with an obstacle in meditation. For instance, your back hurts. That's always a good one. You're sitting and you think you've gotten yourself really comfortable. You think, *I'm going to sit for fifteen minutes without moving.*

Then your body says, *Oh, yeah? That's what you think! Okay, back, do your job: Start to hurt and distract her.*

So the obedient back goes toward an Academy Award for Best Performance by an Aching Back. Trying to ignore it we think, *I'm focusing on* [whatever your meditation technique is]. *I hear the back calling, but I'm not going to pay any attention to it.* That is the first step.

A child might go away at this point, but most of the time, they're more tenacious than that. Instead of just saying, "Mommy, Mommy," the child will start pulling on you, tugging on you, getting a little louder. At that point, your friend may take a moment and say to you, "Excuse me," turn around to the child, and say, "Not now, honey. I'll talk to you a little later. I'm speaking with Susan right now." She's still calm and she didn't lose too much conversation or awareness; instead she just dealt with the interruption quickly. If you observe the same type of distractions, in your mind, make an agreement with yourself to attend to the *urgent* situation as soon as your meditation is finished. That's the second way you can deal with a distraction.

Some children decide to be very loud and even have a tantrum. (Some backs may decide to do that!) As you're meditating, you feel that the back is still hurting and you say to the back, *Okay, I'll stretch in just a little bit. Then I want you to be quiet after that.* The mind tries to convince you that if you do not move the back, all the blood will stop flowing to it, which will cause permanent damage and you may never be able to sit again. In that case, you realize that the mind will not stop until it has distracted you completely. You can just stop meditating for a moment and briefly stretch, reposition your back or place a pillow in a strategic spot. Make a promise that when you are finished you will rub some oil on it or give it whatever it needs. Then go back to your meditation.

Not all the distractions are physical; some are mental or emotional: "I thought of something and I know that if I don't write it down right this minute it will go out of my mind completely and that million dollars I could make in the stock market will never happen." That's how important the thoughts get in meditation. The stronger they are, the more power they have to distract. Have a pad and pencil beside you and if you get any of these *brilliant* thoughts, as a final resort, just write it down. I would suggest first trying the ignoring stage and the reasoning stage, then, if necessary, jot it down and say, "All right now, mind, go back to the meditation technique." You will find—upon your return after the distraction—that it is more difficult to concentrate. The same thing happens when we are distracted while having a conversation: "Now, where was I?"

Know your mind and be gentle with it. If you have a mind that rebels with "shoulds" and force, use a reward instead of a punishment: "We can take a longer walk later," or "We can spend more time talking to our friend over dinner," or whatever is a healthy reward for you. Don't force it and don't say, "You're going to sit here and you're going to meditate no matter what, young lady. This is good for you!" Most of the time that kind of demand does not work in the long run.

You haven't tried to control the mind for all these years; now suddenly you expect it to behave. Why should it listen to you now? If we would begin to train our minds in the first grade—along with learning how to read and write—the mind and thought waves would be calmer and easier to control now. It is the nature of the mind to be tumultuous and our nature to control it.

Make meditation a good, steady habit. You become well grounded in practice when it is done for a long period of time, regularly and without break and with all earnestness or love.

A long period of time means to do it long enough that it becomes as natural to meditate as it is to talk, walk, and breathe. This is not something easily accomplished in one or two months. Set aside a certain time each day for the practice. Be practical. If you set your goals unrealistically high and cannot fulfill those goals, you feel like a failure. If you set realistic goals, you feel good about meeting them. To begin with, take ten minutes once or twice a day and be true to it. Allow it to become a *good* habit. After a while—maybe in a month or more—if you have kept to the ten minutes regularly, add five more minutes to the practice time, slowly and steadily building a strong structure.

When you sit, make a firm affirmation or intent: I'm going to sit for fifteen minutes every morning and evening. No matter what happens during that time, no matter what I think of as important, I'm going to sit without moving. You can even add a particular time of the day: eight o'clock every morning or six o'clock every evening.

Have each day become a rhythmic, regular meditation routine, a routine that becomes as much a part of your day as getting up and brushing your teeth. Do you think of getting up and going out without brushing your teeth or washing your face? It's not the way most of us were raised. In that same way meditation becomes a good habit. Get up, brush your teeth, wash your face, and meditate. Come back from work, meditate, eat dinner, go to sleep. It becomes a natural progression. If for some reason you don't meditate on a particular day, you may not feel quite right—just like you don't feel clean if you don't brush your teeth or wash your face. One is a cleansing of the body, the other a cleansing of the mind.

Our mind comes up with great excuses for what is regularity. I heard a Yoga teacher tell her students that four or five times a week is enough. In my experience the four or five times becomes three or four times and then one or two fades into zero. "I don't need to do it on my vacation when I am relaxed, do I?" With a less busy schedule, we are able to do *more* on holidays and days off, the opposite of time off for good behavior. More time for meditation helps encourage our best behavior.

What is meant by all earnestness? Some great teachers have called it not earnestness, but a deep *love* for the practice. Remember, when we love something we will do it with our whole heart.

A student of a great teacher once asked what it meant to have all earnestness in his practice . . . what would that feel like? Without speaking, the teacher simply motioned for the student to follow him to the lake. Directing the student to enter the water, the teacher followed. Deeper and deeper they went. Finally, when they were shoulder-deep in water, the teacher placed his hand on the student's head and pushed him under the water. Somewhat relaxed, the student felt trust and excitement, anticipating a secret initiation. After some time, the need for air won out over the other expectation. Flailing arms and legs, the student struggled for that precious breath. He was unable to move. Desperate, the student—with all his might—pushed himself up just as the teacher was pulling him out of the water.

"What," asked the teacher, "were you thinking about while under the water?"

Still gasping for breath, the student exclaimed one word: "Air!"

"Anything else?" the teacher asked.

"Air was the only thing I wanted! It was the only thing I could think of."

"Yes," smiled the teacher, "when you want to know yourself as much as you wanted that air, then you shall have it."

When all three criteria—a long time of practice, regularity, and earnestness—are met, we feel a natural flow with our spirit.

Take a minute after concluding your meditation to send out wishes of peace and joy to the world. Use whatever words you would like; it could be an *official* prayer or an unofficial prayer from the heart. If you think of any people who particularly need good wishes, include them in your thoughts and hold them in your heart. I think of this time like the time directly after watering a plant. If the plant is moved too soon after watering, much of the water spills out. It does not have enough time to seep in. It seems to be the same with meditation. Allow the peace to seep in and water your soul.

Creating a Sacred Place

Create a sacred place in your home that draws you in and inspires you to spend time practicing Yoga and meditation. It can be a corner of a room or if possible an entire room, dedicated to your inner self. Have a special pillow or chair, some blankets, a candle, flowers or plants, inspiring pictures, inspirational books—anything uplifting to encourage you to be still and go within. Each time you pass that place, let it remind you of the peace within you. Most rooms in our homes have specific purposes: The bedroom is for sleeping or resting; the bathroom is for cleansing. We may not feel hungry when we step into the kitchen, yet the vibration of food in the kitchen stimulates our hunger. Seeing and feeling our quiet place can entice us to feel the hunger for peace.

It is best to choose a time of day for the practice when you feel fully awake and when the stomach is light. The food we eat plays an important part in being able to sit comfortably and meditate (more about that in Chapter 7, Eating for Wholeness). Simple, clean, easily digested foods allow the body and mind to be more healthy and peaceful. We eat what we need to maintain a feeling of lightness and health. Heavy food will cause drowsiness and instead of superconsciousness, you will fall into sleep consciousness. Try experimenting with eating a lighter diet using more fruits, vegetables, and grains and notice if it makes a difference in the quality of your practice.

Do not allow the world to permeate your special place. Turn off the ringer on the phone. Do not allow any, even friendly, intruders to enter. Leave all worldly thoughts or worries behind as you open your mind to the peace within.

Preparing the Body for Meditation

Many of us are unaccustomed to sitting still and (at least outwardly) doing nothing. At first when sitting still you may observe aches, pains, and stiffness you never knew were there. It is very helpful to have a regular daily routine of gentle stretching to help alleviate the discomfort (see Chapter 6, Move and Heal—Physical Poses). A little stretching first can make a big difference in your ability to be still. Without a still body, the mind cannot be still.

One often asked question is "Why can't I do meditation in an easy chair or even in bed? Why must I sit with the spine erect?"

We are the connection between the heaven and earth. Through our feet we draw in the earth energy and the heaven energy flows down into the top of our heads. These are energy currents, which flow up from the base of the spine and down again. In order to encourage the upward flow, we sit upright. It's very similar to basic physics: Hot air as energy rises. When we sit on the floor the temperature feels cooler than if we sit on a chair or even stand. In meditation there is a buildup of this particular energy that, if allowed to rise, opens us to places of higher consciousness and awareness. It is from here that our physical, emotional, and mental balance flows. We experience a pleasant distancing from our thoughts, feelings, and even our bodies.

This is all more easily achieved in a sitting position. When lying down for relaxation, we dissipate the energy. We are consciously trying to let go of energy so we can relax. In meditation, we are focusing the energy, raising it up into the heart center (chakra), the throat center (chakra), the brow center (chakra), or the top of the head (crown chakra). Compassion and discrimination are our outward rewards.

Have you ever noticed your posture at a business meeting or a lecture? You may be sitting back in your chair, relaxed. Suddenly the topic changes to something that relates to you directly. Perhaps someone has just offered you a four-million-dollar contract. What happens to your posture?

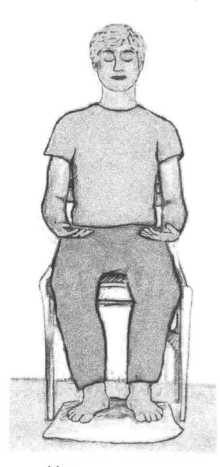

It suddenly straightens. You instinctively know that by sitting upright the energy can flow upward to your brain to allow you to understand, follow, and make the proper comments and judgments. The erect body plays a crucial role in allowing the energy to flow. Form follows function.

If you are seated on a chair, have the feet flat on the floor. If your feet don't touch the floor, you can just move forward until they do or place a pillow under the feet. If comfortable, sit against the wall with the legs outstretched. In this case, have a pillow against the wall supporting the lower back and a pillow under the knees. Many who sit cross-legged on the floor because of photos they have seen quickly realize it is a skill that may take some time to develop. If you choose to sit on the floor cross-legged, have a firm pillow under the buttocks so that the pelvis is tilted slightly forward. For minimizing strain, the knees should always be equal to or lower than the hips in height. (If they are higher, sit on a chair until the body becomes more supple.) You may prefer to sit with your legs under you, feet forming a "seat," or on a meditation bench with the legs folded under. Experiment to see what is most comfortable for you.

Have the arms resting gently on the legs with the palms facing up in a receiving position. When the hands are open

MEDITATION IN A CHAIR

and facing upward we are symbolically putting ourselves in a position to receive. If comfortable, touch the thumb and forefinger together, leaving the three other fingers relaxed in a traditional hand position for meditation called a *mudra*. A mudra is the physical representation of a subtle routing or pattern that helps direct and focus energy. Another traditional mudra is to have the hands resting one over the other in your lap, thumbs touching. When the thumbs in each of the mudras separate, it is a signal that the mind has wandered. By bringing the thumbs back to touch the fingers or each other, the mind is coaxed back into focus.

If these hand positions are not comfortable, just allow the hands to be relaxed. Whichever hand position you choose, be sure that the shoulders are back and relaxed and that the spine remains erect. Have the chin level with the floor and tucked in slightly toward the chest. This brings the neck in alignment with the rest of the spine.

Observe the spine supporting you from the base to the top where the head perfectly balances on its perch. Be aware of each vertebra as it supports and lifts you upward. Since our state of mind is reflected in our bodies and especially in our faces, allow the jaw to be relaxed, the chin level, the face soft with a slight smile. This helps to reflect both inward and outward contentment.

The eyes may be either open or closed. If open, keep them unfocused, resting on a spot in front of you. With the eyes open and still, the focus of the mind is held steady. This is especially useful if you are tired or if the mind is very busy with its thoughts. Having the eyes open allows us to stay focused when meditating.

Having the eyes closed, we can draw deeper within. The eyes are also resting on a spot, this time within. The inner eye rests on the crown (chakra) of the head, the third eye (chakra) between the eyebrows, the heart center (chakra), or the *hara* or *dan tian*—four fingers below the navel (chakra). To have the mind and senses inwardly focused on an energy point or chakra, as suggested above, enhances any meditation technique you are using.

It is interesting to notice that when the mind

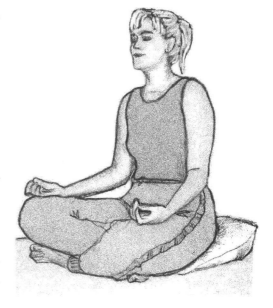

MEDITATION ON THE FLOOR

wanders, the eyes stray from center. As we bring the eyes back to center, the mind follows. In sleep, REM (or rapid eye movements) occur when we are in a dream state. The eyes dart from side to side, accessing thoughts and memories. These same REM occur in our waking mind and also in meditation before the mind is made one-pointed. That is why fixing the gaze can be a great boon for meditators at any stage. In sleep, our minds are unconscious, in waking life conscious, and in meditation supercon-scious—similar appearances, opposite polarities.

There was a study conducted at the University of California, Los Angeles, in the late 1970s that was comparing three of the major medita-tion traditions. The Integral Yoga Institute (IYI) in Los Angeles, where I was director at the time, transcendental meditation (TM), and the Zen center were each to choose ten experienced meditators who had been prac-ticing for at least five years (without a break and hopefully in all earnest-ness). The researchers were trying to discern any differences between the three types of meditations when exposed to external stimulation. Were the meditators really able to draw within so as to not *hear* or *react* to any external noises? In other words, were the subjects in fact meditating?

The TM (repetition of a mantra) and IYI practitioners believed that in *pratyahara* (withdrawal of the senses) the ears would no longer hear and the body would stop reacting to external sounds. The Zen Buddhists claimed that they were ever present and would always hear and react. So let the games begin.

I arrived with some sense of wonder and excitement at the laboratory on my day of "testing." Blanket and pillow in hand, I was asked to sit and do my usual "meditation routine." However, before I began, my body was hooked up to an EEG, a device that measures brain waves. In meditation beta waves normally found in the active mind are replaced by calmer alpha waves and, with deeper practice, even theta waves. I was also wired to an EKG (measuring heart rate and wave fluctuation) and a skin moisture sensitivity test. A set of headphones was placed on my ears and a video camera was keeping a vigilant eye on my every movement.

The researcher left me alone with the instruction to meditate. The lab-oratory theater was *not* the ideal place to practice meditation. The vibra-tion was less than sublime. I transported my mind to a cave in the ancient Himalayas. Holding that image, I spent the next hour doing *pranayama* (breathing practices) and meditating. At an undetermined time I began to hear little clicking noises at what seemed to be regular intervals. The regular became irregular and more and more annoying. At a certain point they faded away.

At the end of an hour, the lights went on and I was released from my wire prison. A worried researcher asked if I was okay. "Yes, I feel great! Is there a problem?"

"At one point," the researcher told me, "your EKG and EEG slowed down to the point of concern. I almost came in and stopped the meditation. I observed you through the camera and you were still sitting upright, so I decided to leave you alone."

Smiling, I asked about the clicking. It seems that even though I thought I had heard the click throughout the entire period, my body and brain stopped reacting after the first few minutes. Even when I found the clicks erratic in time and duration, they were in fact evenly spaced and regular. This seemed to be the consensus with the other two disciplines as well. In fact, according to this study, there was no obvious difference between the three meditation techniques or the experiences of the meditators, once again proof that as quoted in an ancient scripture: "Truth is one. Many are the paths."

PRACTICE OF MEDITATION TECHNIQUES

We are very fortunate in these modern times to have many great meditation techniques available to us. The *best* technique is the one that *suits* you best as long as it is uplifting and enjoyable. Some techniques appeal to the more analytical, cognitive-type person (left side of the brain). Others appeal to more abstract, intuitive-type persons (right side of the brain). There are some that appeal to both sides. Choose for yourself, not from popularity or convenience. There are many methods that are tried-and-true and have been used for thousands of years as they have a certain power associated with them, a buildup of energy. You may choose to take the superhighway (the tried-and-true) and later switch to a footpath (your own way).

Of the many valuable meditation techniques, I will describe a few. Each can be done separately or combined together. It is important to use the one that suits your temperament the best.

Stay with your technique and allow it to take you to a deep state of meditation. Once that state is reached, leave the technique and enter dynamic stillness.

The Eye of the Beholder

Gazing, or *tradak,* is a wonderful technique for people starting in meditation or for those days when the mind is overly active. It is the main technique I have used when working with children. This starts with an external object and then draws us inward. The restless mind is allowed to observe something real, concrete. We use the outward and inward vision alternately; this keeps the eyes and the brain working together. Choose any object you like that will inspire you. It could be the delicate beauty of a flower or a simple candle flame, a photograph, a mandala or yantra (geometric design), a sunset—anything that allows you to feel quiet and peaceful.

Each evening after a very stressful day working at a medical clinic, I joined hundreds of other people in making a pilgrimage to watch the sunset at the ocean. We would leave our cars and worries in the parking lot and jog to a front row seat on the rocks or on the beach. For several minutes we seemed to be united in body and mind, sitting in stillness and gazing at this daily miracle of beauty. After the last ray had dissolved into the sea, leading us into another night, the unity of the gazers would begin to fragment. Some would continue to sit and others would walk, jog, or slowly meander back to their cars (minus the worries). For many, it had become a nightly ritual for meditation and releasing tensions.

Like the setting sun, an inspirational object is placed directly in front of you at eye level close enough for you to see the form and get the feeling. It is not necessary to distinguish details. Glasses or contact lenses are removed so that the eyes are able to relax and soften.

Practice of Gazing Meditation

 Have the body in a comfortable position—either in a chair with the feet flat on the floor or cross-legged on the floor. Have the spine erect, shoulders back, not leaning to one side or another, forward or back. Begin to observe the body. Check to see if the toes are relaxed, then the feet, ankles, shins and calves, knees, thighs, hips, hands, wrists, forearms, and so on.

Inhale through the nose and, as you exhale, let the breath out very slowly, releasing with it any tension that you might feel. Take in another breath and let it out even more slowly. Feel yourself relaxing. It is important to repeat this breath and release tension anytime you feel it starting to seep into the body and mind.

Allow the eyes to close and the body to be still. Slowly open the eyes a little more than halfway. Keep the eyelids relaxed, soft. At first, the eyes will wander. Gently begin to gaze at the object you have chosen and follow the qualities of the object as you go deep within. Keep the eyes open until they blink, tear, or feel any discomfort. Close them softly and allow them to rest. Observe the image as it appears in the mind's eye. When that inner image begins to fade, open the eyes again and gaze at the external object. Repeat this sequence several times.

If the mind starts to wander and brings in stories about the object, gently bring your attention back to the object in front of you.

Keep the breath normal, breathing through the nose. Resist the temptation to reach out and grasp the image with your vision. Instead, allow the eyes to be soft, the image to flow in.

Now imagine how the image might feel—its warmth, coolness, texture, beauty, or simplicity.

Continue the process, gazing outward and gazing inward. See if you can let all the thoughts and feelings go and just concentrate on your chosen object of meditation. If you begin to feel any tension in the body, take in a few deep breaths and let it go.

Allow the eyes to close. See the image with the inner eye as you draw deep within for a more internal meditation. Be still for a few minutes and enjoy the inner tranquility.

Keeping the eyes closed, slowly and gently bring the hands together and briskly rub the palms together, generating heat. When you feel a warmth from the hands, take the palms and gently cup them over the eyes. Allow the darkness and the warmth from the palms to penetrate deep into the eyes and behind them, soothing away any tension you might feel. Very slowly bring the fingertips down and stroke the eyelids out toward the ears, removing any tension or strain from the eyes. Then return the hands to the lap. Relax. Stretch out the body. Observe how peaceful and centered you feel.

The Breath of Life

For the next meditation technique, we observe the breath and begin to join the outer world with the inner world. As the waves gently come onto the earth and return to the sea, so our breath enters the body and then returns to the world. Our breath naturally flows in and out about sixteen times a minute, back and forth, in and out, gently and evenly. We often use the word *inspiration* to mean something that comes to us from a higher place. To inspire is also to breathe in. To expire is to leave the body, to let go and to exhale.

The rhythm of the breath is a wonderful and relaxing way to engage the mind. Many of us have sat for hours listening and watching the waves crashing on the shore. We now have the opportunity to observe the body's tide—the breath, which affirms life as it comes in and encourages us to let go and trust as it leaves. We can observe the coolness of the breath as it comes into the body and the warmth as it leaves. Experience the expansion and contraction of the belly, how the entire body seems to move in unison with the breath. We draw in from the world with the inhalation and on the exhalation we return a little bit of ourselves.

As we sit quietly observing the breath we feel a oneness with the entire creation. We breathe the breath of every living thing. Rich or poor, good or bad, the breath comes in and out. You may find that judgment begins to fade and is replaced by an openness, an acceptance of the perfection of life's flow. Continue to focus on the rhythm of the breath. This connects you with the rhythm of your own heart, a flow with the ocean of life.

Being an ancient practice, this technique is also seen in the Buddhist tradition.

A young student was asking a master what to expect after years of practice. He wanted to make sure it was *worth his while.*

"If I begin to observe my breath what will happen in two years?"

"You will watch your breath," replied the ancient priest.

"What if I watch my breath for ten years, what will happen?"

"You will watch your breath," replied the ancient priest.

"And after fifty years, then what?"

"Ahh!" said the priest, with a big smile. "After fifty years you and the breath will watch each other!"

A nice addition to the breath meditation is to observe the sound the breath makes on its inward and outward journey. As you observe the breath, listen. Can you hear the sound as the air comes into the nostrils? Listen closely to the sound as it leaves. Do they sound different? You may hear a slight hiss or even the sound *soo* as the breath enters and a slight humming sound, *humm,* as it leaves. Listen to the sounds as the breath enters and leaves. Combining two senses, you are observing the feeling of the breath as well as hearing the sound.

Practice of Breath Meditation

Observe your posture. By now, just thinking about meditation, your back will straighten and your shoulders and arms will come into a comfortable position. Allow your eyes to remain open and unfocused or gently close them. Take in a few deep breaths and let them out slowly. Allow the breath to return to normal, easy and gentle. Observe it as it slowly flows in and out of the nostrils without hesitation or strain—life-affirming breath.

Begin to notice any temperature change at the nostrils. As the breath comes in, it is slightly cool and as the air leaves, it is slightly warm. Observe the coolness and the warmth as it comes and goes. The inbreath continues down into the lungs and causes the chest to expand. Observe the belly as it moves in and out, not controlling the breath in any way. Just observe the flowing in and the flowing out, like the tide, like the gentle waves coming onto the shore, without any hesitation: It comes in and gently rolls out. As you draw the breath into the body from the outer world, feel it expand and then, as you send your warm breath back into the world, the body contracts slightly. Allow the mind to focus gently on the movement of the breath.

The whole body seems to move in rhythm with the breath. As the air leaves, feel the abdomen and chest release and relax. Continue to observe the natural flow of breath without force or control.

If the mind begins to wander from the breath, gently bring it back to the flow, in and out. Notice how the rest of the body feels. Is there tension?

If you start to lose the sensitivity of the breath, breathe in a little bit deeper. Feel that coolness and alternating warmth once again.

Notice any outward sounds that might seem further away as you draw inward.

You might even observe a slight smile coming to your face as the body and mind relax and touch that place within you of peace and calmness.

Observe the stillness of the breath. Observe the stillness of the mind and the relationship between the two.

As you are ready to come out of the meditation, slowly begin to increase the inhalation, allowing the outside world to enter your inside world. With the exhalation send a message of peace to all. Allow the eyes to open halfway and see the world in a slightly different way.

In the Beginning Was the Word

The word *mantra* has found its way into our common language usage today. It is always amusing for me to open the newspaper and find the word *mantra* in the comics or financial section. They are using it to mean a word that, when spoken, wields its own power. In the ancient Sanskrit language *Man* means "mind," *tra* "to transcend." A mantra is a word, sound, or phrase that, when repeated, allows us to transcend the thoughts, mind, and our ordinary view of the world. The constant repetition of a mantra is called *japa*.

These inspiring words or sounds can come from many traditions, old and new. Those found in holy books or ancient languages have a certain uplifting vibrational quality. With these words, it is not *just* the meaning but a very special quality that has vibrated from the beginning of time.

The repetition of a word or prayer shows strongly in the Roman Catholic tradition with the rosary. In Russian Orthodoxy, they are encouraged to repeat the Lord Jesus prayer constantly. In the Islamic tradition sacred prayers are repeated five times each day. In Judaism the blessings at mealtimes, Sabbath, and sacred holidays are echoed from thousands of years to the present.

The Bible tells us, "In the beginning was the *word* and the word was with God and the word *was* God." Can you feel a special vibrational quality when going into an ancient place of worship? The sound vibration is palpable. Just by sitting in a temple or church, our minds and hearts are immediately uplifted. We are able to feel many thousands of devoted prayers charging the atmosphere with healing vibrations. Even if you are not religious, it is difficult to deny the comfort that can be drawn from such a place.

Words or prayers in ancient languages can be especially powerful when repeated with mind and heart. In Sanskrit *Om,* the universal consciousness, is chanted as the sound from which all other sounds resonate. *Shanthi* vibrates a feeling of peace. *Om shanthi* then becomes the universal consciousness as peace. From the Hebrew, *shalom* also vibrates a very deep feeling of peace. Notice how *Om shanthi* and *shal-om,* are similar in sound and even in meaning. In the Christian tradition, prayers to Lord Jesus and Mother Mary, *Ave Maria,* are repeated with devotion as is the final *amen. Om, amen,* and *ameen* are words that seem to unite us in sound and vibration even if the traditions are diverse.

The idea of universal consciousness in sound may not always resonate to the nonbeliever. One nonbeliever I met, a nuclear physicist, was working on his neutron accelerator (a neutron smasher) at a major university. I had the occasion to stay at his home, when his wife, a Yoga teacher, invited me to give a talk at the university. After the evening event, the scientist and I exchanged many questions. At first it seemed as if we were speaking very different languages, although we both spoke English. I was fascinated by advanced physics, even though I could not pass Physics 101!

He told me that a probe in the far reaches of the universe had just sent back a sound. This was a surprise to scientists at that time. Most expected the emptiness of space also to be void of any sound. The sound, when described to me, put a smile on my face. It was the cosmic hum or the om sound!

Science and spirituality are only at opposite ends of the spectrum if the spectrum is linear. A circular pattern puts the two "ends" right next to each other! In the beginning, middle, and always is the sound or word.

We are very much a verbal society, propelled by and working with words. The word, it is said, is mightier than the sword. The old adage "Sticks and stones will break my bones but words will never hurt me" is now known to be untrue. Lawsuits are very prevalent for saying hurtful and untrue words about someone. Yet no one is ever sued for saying nice things about someone. With *japa* we are reminded of the peace within—we hear the word, see it, and say it—and our bodies, minds, and worlds open and reflect that peace.

If ancient words are not to your liking, choose more familiar words such as *one, peace, joy, love,* and the like, words that allow us to feel uplifted. Love goes all over the world. If you wish, put it in French *(amour)* or Italian *(amora).* Choose a word, when repeated, whose feeling vibrates within you. Think how you feel when someone says the words *I love you* and then say it to yourself—one hundred, two hundred times a day.

When we continually repeat *any* word or phrase, the cells in our bodies and minds begin to vibrate with that sound. We take on the *qualities* of that word.

These sounds seem to be used by us at our most vulnerable times. We hear a soft moaning sound coming from a sick child and also from the mother who comforts the child. If we are thoroughly enjoying a meal, we use a very similar sound to express our delight. We also hear the release of a sound in passion when a complete word will not exactly express what we are feeling at that moment.

One of the difficult aspects of life for me was my entrance into the electronic age, especially computers. It was necessary for me to learn how to use one in order to write this book. Each time I made an error, the computer would make an unpleasant reproaching sound that made me feel worse than I already felt. To my relief, with help, I was able to record my own voice saying "I love you." Now, instead of a scolding sound, I hear "I love you" and somehow the mistakes seem much less traumatic. A soothing word works wonders.

Can you think of the words you use every day? Do you have a pet word that may not be as sweet and as loving as it could be? Many of the little irritations of daily life may give you cause to use these particular words all too frequently: I missed that blankety blank phone call, or I didn't get that blankety blank parking space, or turning a block too soon and getting into a blankety blank traffic jam, missing the blankety blank bus, and on and on. Can you remember the last time you banged your toe on the coffee table? Did you say *Om* or peace?

An example of a word that children often use is *yuck.* Suppose we began to use the word *yuck* each time we made a mistake: "Yuck this; yuck that." "Oh, that is yucky!" If you said it two or three hundred times a day, how would you feel by the end of the day? Very yucky!

In the same way, imagine saying *peace* two or three hundred times each day. That simple word would soon steady and uplift the mind and permeate your very being.

"How many times must I say this in order for you to understand what I am saying?" The answer is usually "Many!" Did you ever have to write a certain phrase on the blackboard over and over until you learned the lesson? Repetition in all forms allows us to change the thought waves in our minds.

There are many ways to repeat the word. When you are alone, repeat it aloud in a monotone or even a singsong or chanting fashion. Say it softly, loudly, quickly, or slowly, depending on how the mind and emotion feel. Meet the mind where it is.

The ancient ritual of chanting uses a word or phrase sung over and over again. When we sing or chant both sides of the brain are engaged. The left repeats the word as language and the right enjoys the melody or tune. It has been passed down for thousands of years. Chanting in the original ancient languages can still be heard on the holiest of days in each religion. It also seems to have modern significance.

Because of its remote location, a Catholic monastery on a small island off the coast of Italy was able to keep many of its ancient traditions. In this particular monastery Gregorian chanting had been done for countless centuries. Each new fledgling monk was carefully taught pronunciation and tone. Many hours a day were spent in chanting and prayer.

When the new abbot was installed he felt that *too much time* was being taken up in prayer and meditation. If the monks shortened the time in chanting, more productive work could be done. After a few months, the monks started to fall ill. Some were unable to sleep and productivity started to plummet. The water and food sources were examined. All were found to be pure. "What could be the problem?" the senior monks pondered. Physicians were called in from far and wide to no avail.

As a last resort, an expert from America was summoned. He was researching the effects that energy from sound and chanting had on the physical body and mind. A careful assessment was taken of the situation. He then gave his recommendations: Allow the monks to go back to their original scheduled hours of chanting. Their bodies and minds have been toned to a particular frequency, which allows them health and vitality.

They will then be able to do more productive service in less time.

The chanting was restored and so was the health of the monks. It was later suggested by the research findings that this type of chanting was so powerful that even playing a *recording* in the background while working could elicit a calm and healing vibration. I am sure the same could be said for all of the chanting in ancient languages.

In workshops and classes, I often begin by asking everyone to chant *Om* together. At first, people are reluctant to chant, but after experiencing the uniting vibration, more join in. Even if you do not have a "good" voice, try chanting or singing a simple inspirational song softly to yourself. It will usually have such a calm and soothing effect that you will enjoy it often.

When you have become accustomed to the sound and vibration, permit the lips and tongue to repeat the word nonverbally, delicately and thoughtfully, in a silent whisper.

Moving further in, let the mind repeat it in silence, the vibration touching each cell, the whole being vibrating as one sound. All the cells align in the same direction, drawing that peace to you, like iron filings to a magnet.

After a while, with steady practice the mantra may begin to repeat itself. Just sit and listen and enjoy it. This is called *ajapa,* "without repetition." As you move further away from the thoughts, the mind may become very still, so still that it does not even want to *repeat* the word. Just let the word or any other technique drift away. And when you're quiet, just be quiet. Enjoy the peace. The goal has been achieved.

Practice of Mantra Meditation

Choose a word or phrase that inspires you. Adjust your body so it is comfortable. Allow the eyes to close or have them half closed, gazing downward. Inhale and on the exhalation, slowly repeat aloud your chosen word. Continue the repetition with each exhalation. Repeat it over and over, like a wheel turning round and round. With each repetition move further toward the stillness at the center of the wheel.

Inhale and with the exhalation, repeat the sacred word. Begin to say it with the voice—a *gentle whisper,* as if you were speaking to your beloved inside the heart, inside the mind. Allow the voice to become quieter, gentler.

Now allow only the *lips to move,* to repeat the word without any audible sound. Allow the lips to repeat the word with silent reverence. Let it permeate each cell and thought in the body and mind. Have your full awareness on each repetition.

Begin to *repeat silently* the special word you have chosen. Allow the lips to be still and continue the repetition with the mind and heart.

Combine the word with the inbreath. Hear the word whispered as the breath comes in and fills you. As the breath leaves the body, allow the word to flow out, to become a wish to the world. Breathe the vibration in and breathe it out.

Keep focused as the mind and heart silently repeat that special word. Let it draw you inward to embrace each part of you in body and mind. Repeat the word until it transforms you from the inside.

As you are ready to come out of the meditation, slowly and gently begin to take in a deep inhalation. Hear the power of your word coming in, feel the vibration. On the exhalation, in a whisper, softly send the word out as a wish to the world.

Slowly and gently allow the eyes to open halfway. Become aware that you are deeply within, looking out through the windows of the soul.

Writing Meditation

When sitting to meditate, if you find the mind is very agitated, *likhet japa,* or writing of the mantra or word, can be just what is needed. Being placed on hold on the telephone can be very irritating, but mantra writing can be very productive. Notice, to your delight, that when the person returns, instead of being annoyed for being kept waiting, you feel clear and ready to meet the next challenge.

Keep a special notebook or a fresh piece of paper handy. Begin to write and form the letters of the word, saying and feeling each sound. As the hand becomes occupied the mind quiets. This is especially effective if the word you have chosen does not have an everyday meaning for you. If you are artistic, try using the words to form a picture or design, even using different colors. Have a period of stillness at the end. Observe the balance of mind and body.

Walking Meditation

Sometimes the body is not comfortable sitting for a long period of time. Sitting meditation can be alternated with walking meditation.

Begin to walk, taking slow, deliberate steps. Have the hands behind your back. Observe how you place your feet on the floor. Notice the entire body shifting its weight. When the slow walking is in progress, coordinate the inhalation with the placement of the right foot on the floor. The exhalation comes as the left foot lands on the floor, the inhalation as you place the right. If your steps are very slow, inhale as you raise the foot; exhale as the same foot is grounded.

A mantra or word can also be used with walking meditation. Each time you step with the right foot repeat the word. Each time you step with the left foot repeat the word, establishing a rhythm. If you find that your foot and breath have moved out of synchronicity, it means the mind has wandered.

In walking, the mind and the body stay united. The right and left sides of the brain function as one; neither is dominant. We are thinking and acting in balance. When we come back to sitting meditation, the balancing effect is dramatically felt. Some have told me they were unable to meditate until they tried this walking meditation.

This is a wonderful adjunct to any sitting meditation. You can even use it walking from the car or bus on the way to and from work.

Self-Inquiry—Analyzing Meditation

This meditation technique engages the mind to challenge the mind. With the same inquisitiveness that we use looking outward, we can look inward. When we observe a small child between the ages of two and four, this technique becomes clearer to us. Picking up a flower, the child might ask, "What is this?"

"That's a flower," we are happy to offer.

"What kind of flower?"

"A daisy."

"Where does the daisy come from?" And so the questions continue until you have no answers for the child. Still the questions continue: "Why this color?" "Why is the sky blue?" Finally, it is the adult, not the child, who gives up.

In this form of meditation, the mind asks the mind questions or gives the thoughts in the mind labels: What kind of a thought is this? It is a judging thought. It is a wanting thought. It is an observing thought.

We allow ourselves to be our own witnesses, observing ourselves walking, eating, sitting, working. Each thought becomes a slow observation, not a mindless rush. Even our breath is labeled—"Breath in, breath out." It is the hope that the thinking mind will eventually give up.

I take this ancient meditation practice from the Jnana Yoga, or wisdom tradition. It could easily reflect a number of other wisdom traditions.

Practice of Who Am I? Meditation

Have the body in a comfortable position, spine erect, shoulders relaxed. Begin to observe the body. Check to see if everything is relaxed—the toes, the feet, ankles, shins, calves, knees, thighs, hips, the hands, wrists, forearms, and so on.

Through the nose, inhale and as you exhale, let that breath out very slowly—and with it any tension that you might feel. Take in another breath and let it out even more slowly. Feel yourself relaxing.

Place the sense of *I* in the center of the head.

Ask yourself:

Who am I?

Am I the body? The flesh? The bones? The blood? The organs?

No, I am not the body!

Who am I?

Am I the organs of motion?

Am I the arms that reach out? No, I am not the arms or the action of reaching.

Who am I?

Am I the legs that propel the body to move and touch the earth? No, I am not the legs or the movement of the legs.

Who am I?

Am I the organs of the senses?

Am I the eyes that see all sights? No, I am not the eyes or the seeing.

Who am I?

Am I the ears that hear all sounds? No, I am not the ears or the hearing.

Who am I?

Am I the nose that smells all scents? No, I am not the nose or the smelling.

Who am I?

Am I the tongue that tastes and talks? No, I am not the tongue or the sense of taste or the action of speech.

Who am I?

Am I the skin, the sense of feeling? No, I am not the skin or the sense of touch.

Who am I?

Observe and experience your sense of:

> the eyes and inner and outer seeing
> the ears and inner and outer hearing
> the nose and inner and outer smells
> the tongue and inner and outer tasting
> the tongue and inner and outer talking

Who am I?

Am I the mind?

No, I am not the mind.

How can I be the mind if I observe the mind? I must be something other than the mind.

Who am I?

Am I the thoughts?

No, I am not the thoughts because I can observe and change the thoughts.

Who am I?

Even the original *I* that was put in the center of the head is not me because I put it there.

Who am I?

I am beyond all these things. I am Absolute Truth, Absolute Knowledge, Absolute Bliss.

Who am I?

I am the one who knows.

"THE MAN WHO

HAS NO INNER

LIFE IS THE SLAVE

OF HIS

SURROUNDINGS."

—Henri Frederic
Amiel

CHAPTER 6

Move and Heal—Physical Poses

WHEN I FIRST BEGAN TALKING about Yoga some thirty years ago, many people confused it with the white dairy product that is mixed with fruit, yogurt. Over the years, the public's sophistication grew until people now understand—through many great books and teachers—that there is an ancient discipline called Yoga.

Starting in the early 1960s, more people in the United States became interested in keeping their bodies fit. As the different options for this fitness arose, the practice of the physical aspect of Yoga became popular in the West.

Yoga, with its eight limbs, became well known by the system of Hatha Yoga (*ha,* "sun"; *tha,* "moon"). *Hatha* is the balance of energy between lightness and darkness, sun and moon, masculine and feminine. Hatha Yoga consists of physical poses (asanas), relaxation, withdrawal of the senses (*pratyahara),* and breathing practices (*pranayama).* Of all these practices, the physical postures (asanas) were isolated and became popular. Most people commonly refer to the yoga poses, not the total system, as Yoga.

In the *Yoga Sutras of Patanjali,* the definition of asana is a steady, com-

> "IF ANYTHING IS SACRED, THE HUMAN BODY IS SACRED."
>
> —*Walt Whitman*

fortable pose. Actually, the word *sukha,* most often translated as "comfortable," could also be translated as "happy." The benefit of the poses is to make the body feel steady and happy. When the body is in this state, it leads to a steady and happy mind.

There are many ways of doing yoga poses. Some are gentle, some are strengthening, and some are even strenuous. The yoga poses presented here are very gentle. They are adapted and modified for people who wish to relieve stress, relax, be revitalized, and heal.

The movements are often referred to as poses rather than stretches to emphasize that they are done very slowly and held steady. More intense stretching in an attempt to force your muscles to lengthen may actually make the tension worse as the muscles recoil.

What makes yoga stretching different from most exercise is the *additional* benefit to the internal organs, glands, and nervous and cardiovascular systems. There are poses particularly beneficial to the endocrine glands, the organs of digestion and elimination and sexual function. There is special emphasis placed on the spine and the freedom of energy to flow up and down it. Yoga poses work from the inside out.

Millions of Americans today complain of simple back pain. Perhaps our bodies were not made to sit in chairs—at least not for long periods of time. When we get concentrated or even "relaxed" in our easy chairs, we forget about our bodies and the position of our spines. Many of us sit on our storehouse of energy in the sacrum (sacred). This stops the energy from flowing. We may begin with the spine erect in the morning, but by the end of a long day, we may look like gravity has won the battle. By allowing the back to straighten and strengthen, we can again look to the stars instead of only looking at the earth. Our thoughts and ideas will be elevated, and our thinking will be clearer and more balanced. The spine is also a very important river through which much of our energy flows. By having the back bent, even slightly, the flow of energy is inhibited.

Western science is now discovering what yogis have known for thousands of years: The body, mind, and spirit are not separate. Even speaking about the body-mind connection is not entirely correct. It is not possible to separate them except in theory. Think of the body, mind, and spirit like H_2O. There can be solid (ice), liquid (water), or vapor (air). It is all the same, just different forms that determine the closeness and speed of the molecules. The body is solid (the molecules are closer and slower in movement); the mind is liquid (farther apart and with accelerated movement); while the spirit is air (expanded and boundless). Yet they are all one. Only the forms are different.

In the practice of Hatha Yoga the body, mind, and breath all function together. The mind first moves the energy and then the physical body follows. Meditative movements bring great healing benefits to the physical body and the subtle, or energy, body. This energy body contains the pathways or meridians used in acupuncture. It runs through and around the physical body like a river, carrying energy to the entire body and mind. The postures are designed to move the energy through these same pathways by various bending and stretching movements.

This is the same premise used in many of the other spiritual practices that engage the physical body, such as tai chi, karate, or qigong.

A friend of mine, considered a master in tai chi, taught many students the great and ancient art of meditative movement. In order to allow the students the benefit of seeing the roots of tai chi, he arranged a trip to China. They traveled to a remote part of the interior of China to experience the teachings of a great tai chi master.

The morning after their long journey, they eagerly assembled in the front yard for their practice. Feeling the vibration of the *land* of tai chi, they were more concentrated than ever. A small group of people from the local village, hearing of the Americans' arrival, came to watch. For the next three mornings the group of onlookers grew in size. The quiet laughter of the few became more obvious as the size of the group increased. Since none of the spectators spoke English and no one in the American group spoke Chinese, no other communication was exchanged. Finally, by the third day, my baffled friend found a translator.

"Why are they laughing?" the tai chi teacher asked.

"They want to know what the group is doing. Is it some sort of a dance?"

"They are practicing tai chi," he said, somewhat embarrassed to have to explain it to the Chinese interpreter.

After that was translated, the soft laughter turned into howls. "Please, tell us what is so funny," said the teacher.

"The people say that your students are just flailing their arms and legs in the air. In tai chi, the arms and legs move with the flow of energy. They see no movement of energy. The body and mind are moving independently, not as one." The translator shook his head. "They have much to learn about tai chi."

Yoga postures are not unlike certain forms of dance, like ballet, or sports, like golf or tennis. In ballet, the moves are done with concentration and grace. First the mind maps out the movement and then the physical arm follows. In golf, the swing is often done many times in the mind before the ball is actually hit. Once the ball is hit, the eye and the mind's energy follow the ball as if to guide it to its destination.

When the mind images the benefits of the poses, the energy moves more easily to those parts. Then we receive maximum benefits from the practice—a relaxed, healthy body and mind.

These poses are done in quiet or with very soft background music so as not to disturb the concentration of the mind on the body and movement. Some people I know actually watch TV while doing poses. Even though they are stretching the muscles and skeletal system, much of the internal and subtle aspects are lost. When we twist, for example, we squeeze the kidneys. Having the mind focused on someone hitting a home run is not helping our kidneys as much as having the mind focused on squeezing them, thus enhancing the benefits of the pose.

Reg, who now does yoga as stress management every day, had a rocky start with his practice. After an angioplasty some years back, he decided to change his lifestyle. He already faithfully did aerobic exercise and was eating a lowfat diet. His challenge was the yoga portion.

Taking the time to do the slow movement and relaxation seemed like a waste of time to Reg. Being an efficient and creative person, he decided to do the yoga poses while on the treadmill to save time and get the benefits of both. One day, he came down at the wrong moment and his knee quickly reminded him that yoga was a practice requiring concentration and awareness. As he related the story I think his pride was hurt worse than his knee. "Now, every morning I get out of bed and get on the floor and *just* do Hatha Yoga." His practice has made his heart healthy and his life happier. To this day, he still practices at least one hour a day with quiet awareness.

Much of our pain, stiffness, and disease is caused by the lack of or a torrent of energy moving through the body and mind. When flowing normally and rhythmically, the breath regulates the movement of the energy through the energy pathways of the body and mind. This adds another dimension to the poses.

Rhythmical breathing coordinated with movement releases blockages and allows energy to flow, relieving pain and healing disease. Always keep the breath normal and through the nose. The inhalation and exhalation help you relax and stretch further. Holding the breath gives our nervous systems a distress signal. This signal is then sent to the organs, the glands, and the muscular system. By breathing rhythmically, we give the message that this is the time to stretch, relax, and heal.

All this stretching leads us to a supple body of health and strength and a body that is able to be active as well as to sit perfectly still. The system of Hatha Yoga came into being because when the ancient yogis tried to sit still for meditation, their bodies ached and lacked strength; they couldn't concentrate. The poses make the body fit for meditation. It indeed takes a certain amount of discipline and physical strength to keep the body in a firm seated position without movement for a half hour or longer!

Once I was asked to give a lecture and demonstration on yoga poses at a local junior high school. I thought it would be inspiring to show them some of the more complicated poses—more complicated than I was capable of, so I asked a friend who was an adept Hatha Yogi to come with me. I spoke and he demonstrated.

All went well until one of the more chipper students yelled to me, "Hey! Why are you just sitting doing nothing? Why don't you do some poses too?" In fact, I had been sitting still, only moving my head, tongue, and arms for forty-five minutes. It was time to move to the next lesson of Yoga.

"I am doing a very difficult pose," I replied and gestured to my seated posture. My comment was met with boos of disbelief. "Okay, then, let's all try it. Just sit in your seats with your feet on the floor. Let's sit still for five full minutes. Okay?"

"Aw, that's easy!" they chided back. After thirty seconds, there were perceptible squirms and after one minute, the wiggles and giggles began. They reluctantly admitted that sitting still was indeed a challenge of Yoga they were not quite ready to take on.

Many of the yoga poses are named for animals. When observed, it seemed the animals knew the secret of moving and stretching their bodies. If you observe your dog or cat, you can notice that they have an automatic stretching routine they do each time they get up from a rest. Slowly and methodically they stretch one side, then the other. The back arches up and down. We can learn many things from animals and from all of nature.

The poses are done gently and held steadily. Hold each stretch only for as long as it feels comfortable for you without any strain. We are aiding the muscular system in its relaxation; at the same time, we are reaching deeper and more subtle parts of the body. Each part of the body is in turn related to a thinking pattern or emotional feeling. By gently moving the body, we can also move the mind to a state of centeredness. First, we teach this lesson to our bodies and then we bring it into our lives.

The neck seems to be one of the areas of the body that becomes tense and stiff during our normal busy lives. Observing the neck, one can see it is really quite a marvel. The vertebrae are smaller than in the back and yet it is expected to support a head that weighs about eleven pounds, that is, eleven pounds of physical weight. Actually, if we consider the mental weight most of us carry around, the head probably weighs about two thousand pounds. Is it any wonder the neck gets stiff and tired?

The neck is a superhighway passing messages from the head to the heart and the heart to the head. When the head and heart agree, the neck is like an open freeway, moving energy along at sixty miles per hour. If the head and heart are at odds, the freeway gets jammed and the neck starts to ache. Ideally our hearts and minds will have equal input so we can make balanced decisions. The neck is then free from tension.

I am always so careful when teaching the neck movements because of the chronic stiffness most of us carry around. One of my less flexible students came up to me about midway through the twelve sessions. "Did you know that I have had chronic neck pain for many years?" A little nervous, I admitted that I did know that. "I have been to many doctors, massage therapists, and so forth," he said with eyes filming over with tears. I hoped the next thing he said would not be that the neck movements were causing more pain! "This is the first time I can remember that for more than two days in a row I have no pain." So simple, yet so effective.

Neck movements can be done in varied situations—at the office, in a car or airplane—anytime you feel tension starting to build up. When doing the stretches, notice if one side or the other feels stiffer or more relaxed. Reflect on how you use that side of the body. If you work at a computer, is the screen at the correct height? Do you hold the phone between your neck and shoulder? Try to stop, stretch, and move the neck at least once an hour. Notice your mind and senses becoming clearer.

The eyes, also located in the head, are our main information gatherer. We use our eyes constantly during the daytime for work and play. Keeping them focused and fixed for long periods of time on a computer screen, a highway, the television, reading a book or newspaper, or even watching a tennis or golf game causes strain. This also limits our peripheral vision; some of the muscles in the eyes become strong and others lose their integrity. At night our closed eyes move back and forth processing thoughts, looking and searching within.

When we gently and regularly move the eyes in all directions giving them a gentle massage, the six muscles that hold and allow the eyes to move in specific directions are strengthened. You might find that there is an improvement in your eyesight. In some cases, the use of glasses can be dramatically reduced. Even the effects of aging can be lessened with these simple movements. It is one of the easy stress management techniques that can be done at your desk.

A friend of mine was enveloped in a term paper at school. He worked at the computer straight for fourteen hours with almost no breaks. As he was driving home that night he found he was unable to keep his eyelids open to see. This is a *real* problem if you are the driver. He had stressed the muscles so much that they refused to work any longer. Be kind to your eyes and they will be your faithful servants for a long time.

Many of our headaches are caused by neck and eye strain and most of the time we are totally unaware of the abuse.

Those heavy mental burdens that we carry on our shoulders cause much tension and we are chronically hunched over. Also, we tend to cave in our chests as if to protect our hearts from emotional pain. We are protecting them so much that we stop the love from flowing in and out. As we relax our shoulders, we can lay down our burdens and our chest and heart are able to expand.

A series of backward bending poses, followed by forward bending poses, followed by twists help to strengthen and remove built-up tension and correct body posture. When the entire spine is stretched and twisted, it promotes flexibility.

With this series many of the organs in the abdomen are squeezed and revitalized. The pancreas as well as the small and large intestine are replenished with fresh blood and energy. The kidneys and adrenal glands, which are located on the back under the lower rib cage, seem to really enjoy these poses. I picture the kidneys with smiles and the adrenal glands being charged like a car battery on a cold winter's day. In our stressful lives, these organs and glands are adversely affected.

When our adrenal glands run out of energy about 10:00 A.M. or 3:00 P.M., instead of taking a rest or doing some revitalizing poses, what do we do? We jolt them with a cup of coffee. That lasts until the caffeine rush is over, then we are back at the same slump. So another cup of coffee is administered until at last, when we go to sleep for rest and rejuvenation, we are all wired up. You may even want to try a few of these poses at your desk for a healthy boost of energy midmorning or midafternoon.

As we move the body in the poses the head and heart usually go in the same direction, sometimes even in a different direction from the limbs. This could be a metaphor for our daily lives. When we align the heart and head—no matter what the rest of the body or the world says or does—we are in agreement with ourselves.

The inverted poses have many great benefits, both physically and emotionally.

The heart pumps the blood into the arteries, which nourish the entire body. The muscular arteries, with the help of gravity, deliver the blood to the fingers and toes. Getting the blood back up from the feet to the lungs is a greater challenge. The blood returns to the heart via the lungs by veins, which do not have muscles of their own. The blood is pumped upward through the veins by the contraction of the external muscles in the leg. Stop valves at regular intervals keep the blood from draining back down the leg under the force of gravity. Sometimes swelling occurs and even varicose veins (the breakdown of the valves that causes a bulging of the vein). Many of us sit or stand for hours with our feet down. The pull of gravity and lack of muscle movement encourages the blood to pool in our feet and legs. Normal daily walking and exercise assist the return flow of blood.

Varicose veins also occur in areas other than the legs, such as the rectum in the form of hemorrhoids, which are aggravated by constant sitting. All these problems can be helped by good venous return to the lungs and heart.

The shoulder stand aids the return of the blood to the lungs for oxygenation by raising the feet, legs, and pelvis higher than the head.

When I first started teaching the shoulder stand to heart patients there was a concern about the safety of this pose because of the heart's lessened ability to pump blood *up* to the legs. As long as the brain was receiving fresh oxygenated blood the heart seemed to be contented and did not struggle and try to pump the blood up to the legs. We found that the inversion of the legs actually *allowed the heart to rest.* The poor circulation in their legs was also greatly improved with reverse gravity. Reversing the flow of energy also brought about a sense of well-being. The smiles and their reluctance to come out of the pose was all the affirmation we needed that it was bringing benefit.

The lymphatic system is part of the immune system and plays a major role in the body's defense against infection and cancer. Since the lymph system does not have a central pump, lymph is circulated by movement of the muscular-skeletal system in a process analogous to the venous system. Gravity assists the downward movement. Healthy lymphatic vessels are equipped with one-way valves to aid the upward movement of lymph through the body. The shoulder stand and body inversion encourage the return of lymph from the lower extremities. This enhances a healthy immune function.

The shoulder stand also brings great benefit to the thyroid gland at the base of the throat, a butterfly-shaped gland that controls the body's metabolism. While the body is inverted, the throat is gently pressed to the chest. The spongy thyroid gland is squeezed and when it's released fresh new blood rushes in and revitalizes it, helping to balance its function.

Fish pose is one of the inverted poses. Unlike the shoulder stand where the entire body is inverted, here only the head, neck, and chest are inverted. The throat and chest expand as they arch back, allowing the head to tilt backward with the top of the head toward the floor. This pose helps distribute oxygen to the apex (uppermost point) of the lungs. The backward arch of the throat allows the released thyroid gland to infuse with fresh blood and vitality. The concave chest expands, allowing the heart to blossom. This complements the shoulder stand.

The next time you are upset or get disillusioned with the world, try an inverted pose and look at the world from a different angle. Everything looks different and perhaps a little less threatening upside down.

A sense of balance of the body, mind, and spirit is felt with the completion of the poses. The result is that we feel better, look better, and can direct that feeling into the world to do better. When we feel this, no explanation is necessary, but many continue to try to explain it.

By following this simple set of postures on a daily basis, we may find our digestion and blood circulation improve, senses and thinking become clearer, metabolism and glandular system balance, enabling us to control our weight, and, best of all, we may look and feel younger and healthier and thus have a renewed joy for life.

Setting the Stage for Poses

The time of day for practice can be determined by the busyness of our schedule. Early morning seems to work well for many because the day's activities are not yet in full force. The mind is calmer and the lists for the day have not yet begun. Having the recommended empty stomach for the practice is also easier at this time. The poses may look better later in the day, yet the effect of doing them earlier can actually help rid our bodies of the lactic acid buildup that causes early morning stiffness. The day seems to go smoother when we start off relaxed and limber.

Choose a quiet space for the practice. Turn off the ringer on the phone and, if necessary, put a QUIET TIME IN PRACTICE sign on the door. Have a well-padded floor for maximum comfort. If you are not feeling well, many of these poses can be done on your bed.

The temperature of the room should be warm—not too hot or cold— just right for your body to be able to let go. Have at least two pillows and blankets available to use as props and covers.

If you live in a noisy area or there are distractions in your home, a nice music tape helps you to bring the focus inward. Using an instructional Yoga tape (*Relax, Move & Heal,* from the Abundant Well-Being series) encourages you to do the complete session with rests in between. The mind can relax, knowing the tape is the timekeeper. As you become accustomed to the poses and the sequence, you may be tempted to leave out the resting time in between the poses; don't. This time in between the poses is just as important as the poses themselves.

PRACTICE OF THE POSES

These poses are recommended for people of any age and most health conditions. It is up to you to decide what is comfortable to do and what may cause discomfort. (Remember, first, do no harm.) If you have any serious or chronic conditions and question the safety of doing *any* of these poses, please check with your medical practitioner first. Always be slow and gentle so you can anticipate any problem *before* it arises. If at any point you feel real *PAIN, discontinue the pose, relax completely in the relaxation pose, and breathe deeply.* As the pain subsides *you* can decide whether it is best to continue or to finish the session with a long deep relaxation. By doing less you are actually doing more.

Choose a well-balanced basic set as your core poses and vary them as time permits. A good core set for a one-hour practice would begin with a short relaxation, twenty minutes of poses including the neck and shoulder, wrist and ankle movements, one or more backward bending and forward bending, shoulder stand, fish, half spinal twist, and yogic seal.

The sun salutation is always great for an all-body stretch and tone. If you do a lot of work with your eyes, be sure to include the eye movements. The first part, including the relaxation and poses, will take about thirty minutes.

After the poses do a long deep relaxation for fifteen minutes, five minutes of breathing practices, five minutes of imagery (this could be incorporated into relaxation), and finish with five minutes of meditation. This would add another thirty minutes, making the practice balanced and a full hour.

When you feel more comfortable sitting for meditation the physical part can be shortened.

RELAXATION POSE

It is nice to begin the practice with relaxation, which helps us to center and let go of the outside world. It sets the tone for the rest of the practice.

Lie on your back. Have the legs about shoulder width apart, the arms in a comfortable position alongside the body with the palms up, if comfortable, and the eyes and lips closed.

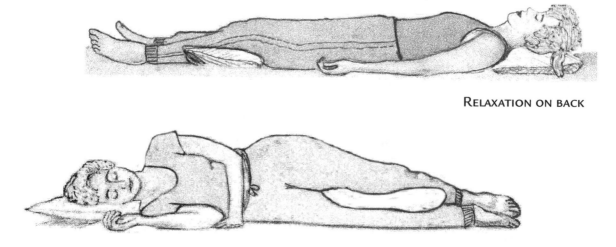

RELAXATION ON BACK

RELAXATION ON SIDE

Place a pillow under your head and knees to allow the back to relax fully and be more comfortable. If on your side, place a pillow under the head and between the knees or sit in a comfortable chair. Take in some deep inhalations and, with the exhalations, release any tension.

Observe the breath as it flows in and out gently through the nose. Using the mind and gentle breathing, relax and remove tension from the toes, feet, legs, and hips, then the fingers, hands, arms, and shoulders. Relaxation manifests as a softening of the limbs, front of the body, and the throat. The back and neck let go and relax as they come closer to the floor. The face becomes smooth; the mind comes into harmony and calmness. There is a stillness and calmness that permeates the body and the mind.

This relaxation pose is done between each of the poses we do on the floor to observe the body and the mind. We are able to pay close attention to what parts of the body are touching the floor. Is there a balance between the right and left sides? Which parts of the body feel heavy and relaxed?

Be aware of any changes throughout the session of poses. If on observation you notice any tension or strain, take in a deep inhalation; imagine a fresh supply of energy entering that part of the body and on the exhalation allow it to relax completely.

Even though this pose may seem simple at first, it is difficult to do for some very active people. The art of this pose is to allow you to feel totally supported so that you are able to let go completely. (Refer to Chapter 3, Deep Rest, Deep Relaxation, for full details.)

When moving from lying on your back to sitting up, always roll over to one side, curl up, and remain there for a few moments. This helps to stabilize the blood pressure, eliminating any dizziness or light-headedness.

NECK MOVEMENTS

We move the neck forward and from side to side. As the vertebrae in the neck are not made as ball joints, it is not recommended to move the head in a circular fashion. Although this circular movement may feel good initially, it can cause long-term problems. Prevention is better than cure.

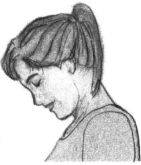

Sit comfortably in a chair or on the floor with your spine erect. Leave the shoulders and arms relaxed. Inhale. Exhale as you bend the head forward so that the chin comes toward the chest.

Breathe normally as you allow all the muscles to relax. With each inhalation and exhalation, feel the gentle stretch on the back of the neck. Allow the weight of the head to help the stretch.

Inhale and bring the head back to the center. Exhale. Relax.

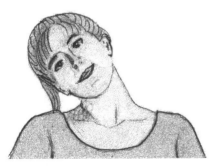

Inhale. Exhale as you slowly bring the right ear toward the right shoulder. Feel the stretch on the left side of the neck. Keep the shoulders relaxed, not raising them toward the ears; just tilt the head toward the shoulder. Keep the breath regular and with each exhalation feel the neck relax. Inhale and raise the head to center; exhale and relax.

Inhale. Exhale as you bring the left ear toward the left shoulder. Relax the head and breathe normally. Feel the right side of the neck relax. Inhale and raise the head back to center; exhale and relax.

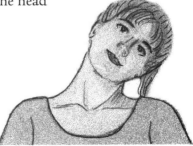

Allow the eyes to close and experience the neck free from tension.

SHOULDER ROTATIONS

In this pose we will make circular movements with the shoulders. Keep the arms and hands relaxed and at your sides so that the weight of the arms aids in the relaxation.

Inhale and slowly begin to raise the shoulders up toward your ears (even further than they already are!); exhale and move them forward as if to touch under the chin. Inhale and bring the shoulders down toward the floor. Exhale and bring the shoulders back behind you so that the shoulder blades come close together. Feel the chest expanding.

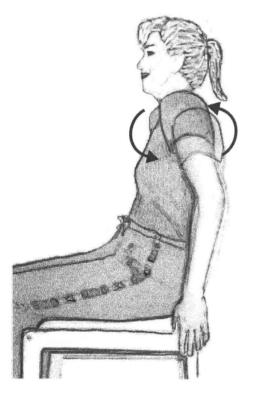

Continue at your own pace. Keep the breath even and moving slowly through each part of the movement. Move even slower through any especially tense or sore spots, coaxing them to let go. After a few repetitions, allow the shoulders to relax. Gently shake the arms.

Repeat the same circular movements in the opposite direction. Keep the breath normal and the arms relaxed. Feel the tension leave the shoulders.

Gently shake the arms and relax with the eyes closed. Notice how relaxed the neck and shoulders feel.

Allow a smile to come to your face as you feel the relaxation and the energy moving freely from the heart to the head and the head to the heart.

All the nerves that nourish the senses run through the neck and shoulders. With tension the flow of energy is inhibited. Without energy the senses dull. Perhaps with the tension gone your senses may be keener, your eyesight brighter, and your hearing clearer. Be still enough to notice any changes.

WRIST ROTATIONS

With all the repetitive work we do with the hands (for example, writing, chopping, computer work) it is important to keep the hands and arms supple and relaxed. Taking a short time each hour can make a big difference in your comfort and flexibility, both physical and emotional.

In a posture reminiscent of hula danc-ing, stretch the arms out and slowly begin to rotate the hands and wrists in a clock-wise direction. Keep the breath regular and the circles small at first. See if you can have both hands going in the same direction. Relax.

Now repeat with a counterclockwise direction. Notice if one side is easier to rotate than the other. Gently shake the hands. Move the fingers in and out of a fist a few times and wiggle them. Relax with the hands open.

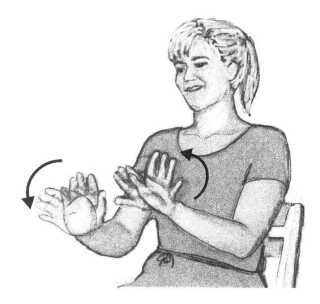

ANKLE ROTATIONS

As we get older, one of the things that happens is that we lose the spring in our step. Our toes and ankles get stiff and the less we move them, the stiffer they get. We spend much of our day sitting or standing and the blood pools in the legs and feet. Simple ankle rotations can help keep the spring in our step.

Sitting on a chair or on the floor, have the legs directly in front of you with the *heels on the floor*. Breathing normally, slowly begin to rotate both ankles by making small circles with the toes in a clockwise direction. Keep the legs still so the movement comes from the ankles, not the legs.

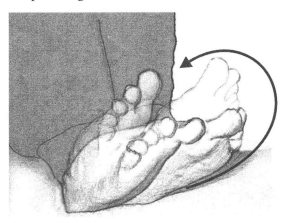

Increase the size of the cir-cles as you feel the ankles relax (three or four times). Relax.

Repeat in a counter-clockwise direction. Gently shake the legs, wiggle the toes, and relax. You may feel a slight tingling as the blood circulates through the feet.

Backward Bending Poses

Lie on your belly, cheek to the side, arms to the side slightly away from the body or on the floor, hands next to the shoulders or head. Have the legs a comfortable distance apart. This is the resting position on the belly. If this is not comfortable, lie on either side with a pillow under the head and between the knees.

The following poses are shown both on the floor and in a chair. Choose which one is best for your comfort level.

COBRA POSE

In this pose we imitate the movement of the cobra, arching up, expanding the chest, and then bending the head majestically back.

Lying on your belly, bring the heels and legs together and keep them relaxed. Palms are flat on the floor beneath the shoulders, fingers pointing forward. Elbows are bent, close in to your body and pointing up toward the ceiling. A slight indentation is felt between the shoulder blades behind the heart. Place the forehead on the floor. (If you are in a chair, have both feet on the floor.)

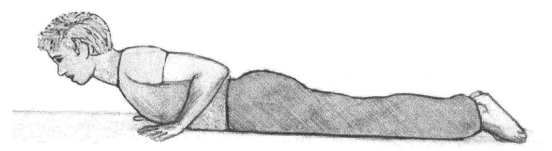

COBRA ON FLOOR

Inhale as you stretch the chin forward. Without pushing down with your hands, slowly raise your head, neck, and chest off the floor, using the upper back. Hands are used for support only.

Exhale, breathe normally, and relax into the pose. Keep your abdomen on the floor and your legs together without any tension. The breath is normal.

COBRA ON CHAIR

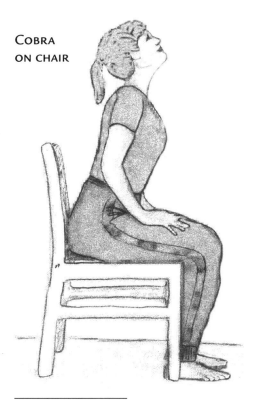

The awareness is between the shoulder blades and on the expansion of the chest and heart center. Hold this pose steady for a few seconds without strain or tension. Be aware to stretch only as far as is comfortable. Each time you do this pose you may have a different capacity.

Inhale, stretch up, and exhale as you slowly roll down in a continuous motion—first touching the chin, then the forehead, to the floor. Turn the cheek to the side; release your arms and legs and relax.

HALF LOCUST POSE

This pose focuses on the lower back, abdomen, and legs. Have both hips flat on the floor and lift each leg off the floor only a few inches.

Lie on your belly with the chin on the floor. Place the arms alongside or tucked underneath your body with the elbows facing each other and your palms up. (If standing, have both hands on the back of a chair.)

Bring the awareness to the right leg. Stretch out the right leg all the way from the hip. Inhale as you slowly raise it a few inches off the floor. Exhale and hold the leg up for a few seconds while breathing normally. Awareness is on the lower back. Notice if you are tensing the buttock or

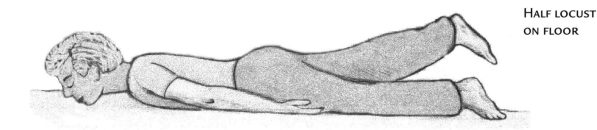

HALF LOCUST ON FLOOR

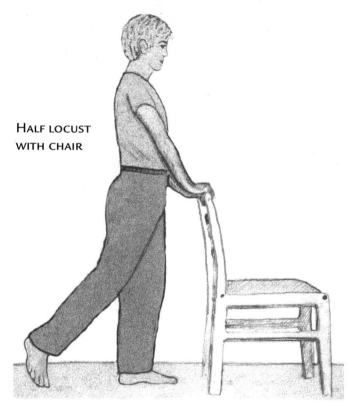

HALF LOCUST
WITH CHAIR

the left leg on the floor in order to keep the right leg raised. If this is happening, lower the right leg until it is supporting itself with help from the lower back.

Slowly lower the leg, then turn the cheek to the side and relax.

Repeat the same sequence with the left leg. Turn the cheek to the side and relax.

Now turn over onto your back and relax completely in the relaxation pose (page 153).

Notice how the upper and lower back feel. Did you stretch too much? Not enough? Just right? Did you lose the breath's normal rhythm? Be conscious of the internal signals. Learn the difference between a good stretch and a stretch that is doing harm.

Forward Bending Poses

Along with stretching the muscles in the back the forward bending poses give a wonderful massage to all the internal organs and help make the spine flexible. In the forward bending poses we must be conscious to actually come forward, not downward. The body moves in the direction the eyes are looking. Pay special attention to the upper chest and heart center and make sure that they are extended and expanded rather than collapsed. These poses teach us to reach forward in our lives and from the heart center.

LEG TO CHEST BENDS

This first forward bend is simple yet very helpful to relieve stiffness in the back. You can even do this pose before you get out of bed in the morning or last thing in the evening. At the office, this pose can be done sitting in a chair (only with one leg at a time).

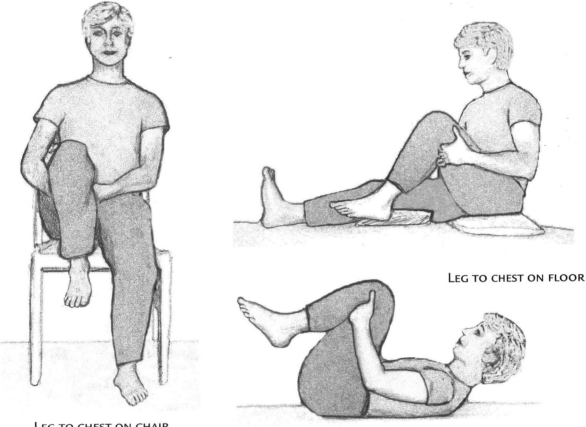

LEG TO CHEST ON FLOOR

LEG TO CHEST ON CHAIR

The leg bends help keep the knees limber and stretch out the lower back, relieving back strain and tension. They help bring a good supply of energy to the pelvic and abdominal organs, allowing them to function normally and effectively.

Best of all, they really feel great, especially after sitting for a long time.

Lying on your back or sitting in a chair, bring the right knee up toward the chest. As you inhale, grasp behind the knee with both hands and exhale, gently bringing the knee closer to the chest. Hold the leg steady. Keep your breathing normal. The awareness is on the lower back.

If you feel comfortable, as the back relaxes, inhale and bring the head toward the knee, giving yourself a gentle hug. Exhale, relaxing the head and breath. Gently place the foot back on the floor. Relax. Repeat with the left leg and, if still comfortable, with both legs at once. Be sure the breath stays even throughout the pose. Relax completely. Notice how relaxed the lower back feels.

FULL FORWARD BEND

In a seated position, have the legs outstretched with a pillow under the knees, the toes pointing up toward the ceiling. (It may be helpful for you to do the forward bend by placing a folded pillow under the buttocks so the hips are tilted forward.) If you are on a chair, allow the feet to rest comfortably on the floor. (If the feet do not touch the floor, place a pillow under the feet.)

Palms together at the heart center, lock the thumbs, stretch the arms out from the heart center, and raise the arms up toward the ceiling. Inhale, stretch up, look up. Exhaling, bend forward, looking at the hands and stretching to the wall in front of you. Inhale and, as you exhale, come forward over the outstretched legs, keeping the back straight and lifting from the base of the spine. Grasp the legs wherever comfortable and allow the head, neck, and shoulders to relax while continuing to keep the chest expanded and the eyes looking forward.

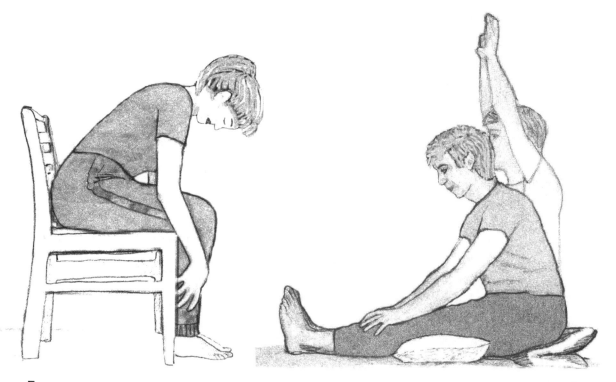

FORWARD BEND ON CHAIR　　　　　FORWARD BEND ON FLOOR

Check to see that there is not *any* discomfort in the legs or back. If there is, please do not come as far forward in this pose. By doing less, you may be doing more for yourself because you are not pushing beyond your present limit and thus creating more tension.

Lock the thumbs and stretch the arms out in front of you. Looking at the hands, come up to a seated position. Slowly bring the arms down with the palms together at the heart center. Relax the arms. Breathe deeply and easily through the nose. Relax completely.

Be aware of any changes in the body. Relax the body and mind completely.

Shoulder Stand

If you have known uncontrolled high blood pressure, diabetes retinopathy, carotid artery disease, or neck problems, please check with a health practitioner before doing this practice. Stage I can often be made comfortable for most people with some minor adjustments.

It is helpful to be on a level, well-padded surface. In Stage I we begin by putting our legs on a chair that is against the wall. When Stage I becomes comfortable, we move to Stage II, using a wall instead of a chair to support the legs. In Stage III we begin to walk up the wall, placing the body in a more vertical position.

Adjust your clothing to loosen any tightness, especially at the neck and throat. Be aware of any dizziness, light-headedness, or discomfort. At the first sign of any of these, come out of the pose immediately and rest in the relaxation pose (page 153).

Ideally we hold this pose for at least three minutes, as this is approximately how long it takes the blood to make one trip through the entire body. The important part is to hold it only as long as is *comfortable for you.*

As you feel more comfortable in the pose, allow your eyes to close for more internal benefit.

The awareness is on the inversion of the body and at the thyroid gland.

STAGE I: SHOULDER STAND MODIFIED WITH A CHAIR

Lie on your back and rest your feet and legs on a sturdy, straight chair that is braced against the wall. Allow the legs—up to the back of the knees—to be resting on the chair, not dangling off. You may need to turn the chair to the side or place a pillow on the edge of the chair to have the legs fully resting on the chair. If the edge of the chair cuts into the legs, it can inhibit circulation.

Place a pillow or blanket under your head and neck, with the folded side supporting the neck. This allows the chin to come forward, putting gentle pressure on the base of the throat and thyroid gland.

Place a second pillow under the buttocks—folded side in—elevating the buttocks and tipping them slightly forward. This allows the blood and energy to flow back from the legs to the upper body.

Allow the breath to be normal. Start by holding the pose for one minute. As you feel more comfortable, the holding time can be gradually increased.

Feel the relaxing and beneficial effects.

Remove the pillows. Slowly bend the knees and place the feet back on the floor. Stretch out the legs, and relax on your back.

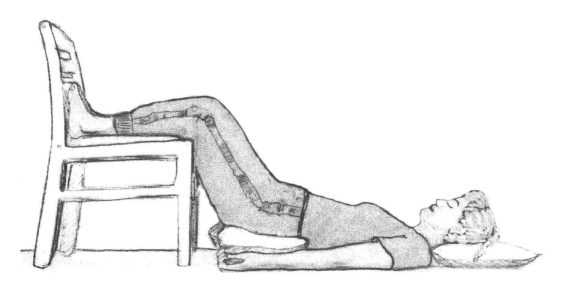

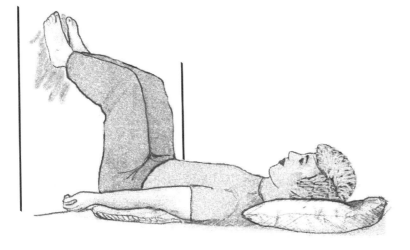

STAGE II: SHOULDER STAND USING A WALL

Use an empty wall for support. Sit on the floor against the wall with the knees bent and the right hip touching the wall. Turn so that you are facing the wall; the buttocks are against the wall (feet are up). Lie back on the floor. Bring the soles of the feet to the wall with the knees bent. Place a pillow under the head and buttocks as in Stage I.

Allow the legs to straighten. Observe any signs of distress in the breath or discomfort in the lower back or chest. If you feel even the beginning of these signs of distress, come out of the pose and rest in the relaxation pose (page 153).

Hold for a minute or longer, as you feel comfortable.

Remove the pillows from the buttocks and head. Stretch out the body and relax on your back in the relaxation pose.

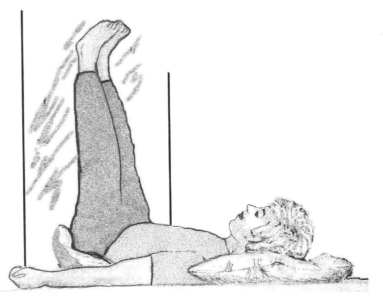

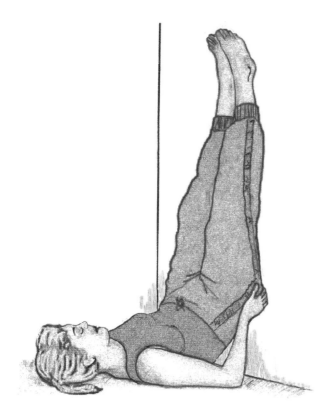

STAGE III: WALKING UP THE WALL

Prepare as in Stage II, this time eliminating the pillows from behind the head, neck, and buttocks.

Begin to walk up the wall with first one foot, then the other. Gently bring the hands to the lower back for support. Go up only as high as is comfortable and steady, straighten the knees, and allow the weight of the body to lean against the wall. The breath is normal.

Hold for a minute or longer, as you feel comfortable.

Slowly begin to walk the feet down the wall and lower the buttocks to the floor. Keep the knees bent until the feet are flat on the floor, stretching out the legs completely. Relax on your back.

Fish Pose

Fish pose is a complementary pose to the shoulder stand in that it gives a reverse stretch to the thyroid gland. All the squeezing that was done to the thyroid gland in shoulder stand is now released, and the blood flows back in like a squeezed-out sponge. We now extend the throat further back to allow maximum absorption.

Another great benefit in this pose is to the chest and lungs. As the chest expands and arches up, the lungs are encouraged to inflate up into the apex, the part tucked under the collarbones.

This pose also helps us correct the chest cave-in posture we acquire from sitting in chairs and from protecting our hearts from emotional pain.

It expresses physically how, when we lead with the heart, the head follows. How strong and powerful we feel when the heart leads!

VERSION I: FISH POSE

As soon after shoulder stand as comfortable, still lying on your back, place a pillow lengthwise between your shoulders. The edge of the pillow should support the neck and base of the head. Allow the neck to bend backward slightly and have the top of the head tip over the edge of the pillow. The heart center and chest are well expanded.

Be conscious of the head tilting back just slightly; go only to your level of comfort.

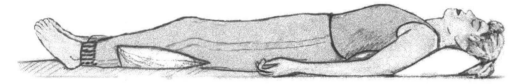

The shoulders are relaxed and expanded. The arms rest at the sides. Place the hands on the floor, legs together and relaxed. Take in deep easy breaths through the nose to expand and relax the chest and to fully oxygenate the system. Allow a soft smile to come to your face.

To come out of the pose, slowly lift the head back to the pillow or remove the pillow from under the head. Rest in the relaxation pose (page 153).

Observe the body for any tension. Release any tension with the exhalation. Feel the benefits of the inverted poses.

VERSION II: FISH POSE

Begin as in Version I. This time have the pillow even with the shoulders. Cushioned by the pillow, allow the head to tip back so that the top of the head is resting on the floor. The heart center and chest are well expanded. Be cautious of any dizziness or light-headedness.

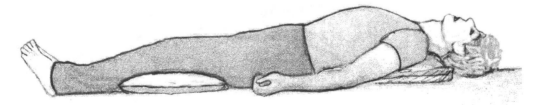

The shoulders are relaxed and expanded. The arms rest at the sides. Take in deep easy breaths through the nose to expand and relax the chest and to fully oxygenate the system. Allow a soft smile to come to your face.

To come out of the pose, gently lift the head back to the pillow or remove the pillow from under the head. Rest in the relaxation pose (page 153).

Observe the body for any tension. Release any tension with the exhalation. Feel the benefits of the inverted poses.

Spinal Twist

HALF SPINAL TWIST

To many people this looks like a "real" yoga pose. Sometimes I refer to it as the pretzel pose.

Sit on a straight-backed chair or on the floor. Cross your right foot over the left leg. If on the floor, have the left leg extended and place the sole of the right foot flat on the floor between the knee and ankle.

Place the right hand on the back of the chair or on the floor behind you close to the body, with the fingers pointing away from the body. With the left hand, press back against the outside of the right knee.

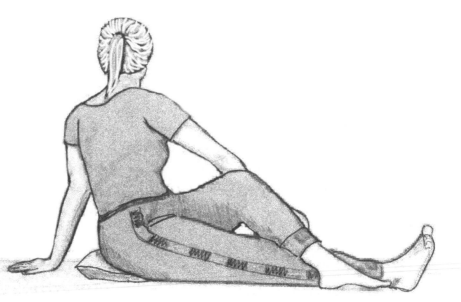

**HALF SPINAL TWIST
ON FLOOR**

Reach toward the left knee or bend the elbow of the right arm and rest it on the right hip. Allow the shoulders to remain relaxed.

Inhale and stretch up. Then exhale, slowly twisting the spine and head around to the right, looking over the right shoulder. Lead with the heart and the head will follow.

Relax into the pose. Breathe normally and easily.

Feel the massage you are giving to all the abdominal organs, especially to the kidneys and adrenal glands.

Inhale. Release the arms and legs; return to center. Exhale and relax. Stretch the arms and legs and give them a gentle shake.

Repeat the same pose on the other side, crossing the left leg over the right and twisting to the left. Remember to breathe!

Notice any difference in the amount of tension or suppleness on the two sides of the body. Can you relate it back to how you use the different sides in your daily life?

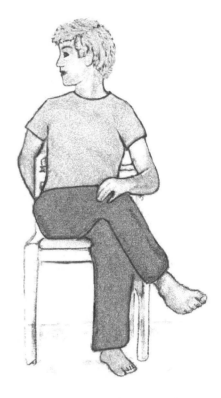

HALF SPINAL TWIST
ON CHAIR

Seal of Yoga

THE SEAL OF YOGA OR YOGA MUDRA

This pose is a wonderful forward bend that has the added benefit of sealing in some of the energy generated by the other poses. Because of this, it is most beneficial to do yoga mudra as your final pose in a series. Some of the great benefits of this pose can be felt by coming up as slowly as possible. When I see people popping up from this pose, I know that much of the benefit cannot be felt. Instead of popping up, when coming out of this pose, feel as if the buoyancy of the lungs is raising you up with each inhalation, as if you are floating up in water. With each exhalation, you may sink back down a few inches, to rise again with the next inhalation. The process could take up to a minute or longer, depending on how close your head is to the floor. When this is done slowly with the eyes closed, you may experience a feeling of deep and profound peace. Sit still for a moment afterward and relish the moment and the feeling.

Sit in a chair or in a comfortable, cross-legged position with the eyes closed.

Bring the arms behind the back and grasp the right wrist. Inhale deeply and stretch up.

On the exhalation, extend the chin. With a straight spine, fold your body forward over the legs, bringing the belly toward the thighs. When you have come forward as much as you comfortably can, allow the body and head to relax with the spine straight.

Inhale deeply as you extend the chin. Slowly allow the buoyancy of the lungs to raise the head and body up with each inhalation. With each exhalation, float down slightly. Continue until you are erect in a sitting position.

Keeping the eyes closed, allow the hands to come to your lap. Sit very still and feel the effect of the yogic seal. Experience the peace within.

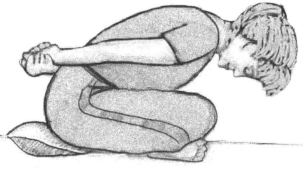

SEAL ON FLOOR

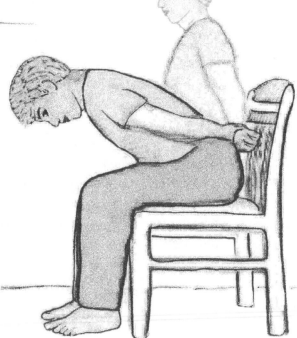

SEAL ON CHAIR

Sun Salutation

This is a series of poses that, when done together, combine many of the benefits of the preceding poses. Sun salutation allows the body to stretch both forward and backward. If done consciously, the body and all of the systems benefit by the intentional stretches. We start slowly and then quicken the speed as the body limbers. It can also be used as a warm-up before or as a cooldown after aerobic exercise. When time is limited, a few rounds can keep us limber until the full set is done.

Since the body is moved up and then down in this sequence, move cautiously to avoid dizziness or light-headedness.

There are three different versions of sun salutation offered here. Try the sitting version first and when that feels comfortable and easeful move to the combined sitting and standing version. As that feels comfortable, the standing version can be done.

Sun salutation is a great way to greet the new day or to stretch anytime during the day. When you are doing these poses, imagine that you are greeting the sun and drawing energy from it to give you strength and healing power. The more you are able to draw inwardly, the more you will be able to discover the sun that is awakening within the center of your being.

The breath is normal and kept even throughout the sequence of poses. If you find the breath becoming irregular, slow the movement or stop and rest.

SUN SALUTATION: SEATED VERSION

This first version is done seated in a straight-backed chair. The feet are flat on the floor or on a pillow on the floor.

POSITION 1: Sit erect, legs together. Bring the palms together in front of the heart center.

POSITION 2: Lock the thumbs. Stretch the arms out from the heart center. Look at the hands as you slowly raise the arms overhead. Stretch from the base of the spine to the tips of the fingers.

POSITION 3: Keeping the arms alongside of the head, look up at the hands and slowly fold forward from the hips. Allow the head to relax toward the legs and the arms to relax toward the floor.

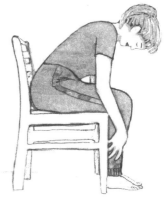

(3)

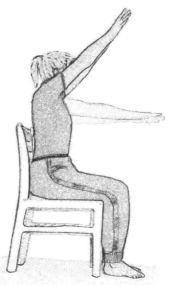

(2)

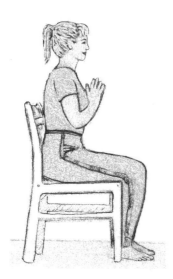

(1 and 12)

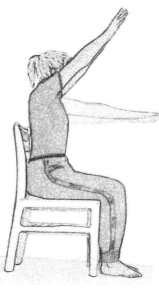

(11)

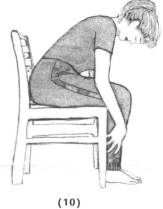

(10)

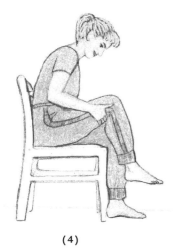

(4)

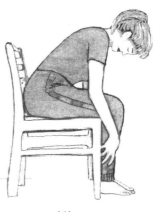

(5)

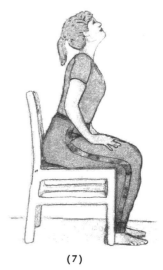

(6)

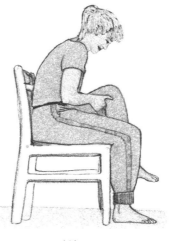

(7)

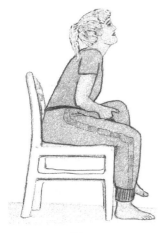

(8)

(9)

POSITION 4: With both hands grasp behind the right knee and lift it up. Bring the abdomen toward the thigh.

POSITION 5: Continue holding the leg, arch the back, bring the shoulders back, and look up.

POSITION 6: Bring the head back to center and release the leg. Stretch out the arms, lock the thumbs, look at the hands, and slowly fold forward from the hips. Allowing the abdomen to come toward the thighs, relax the head and the arms toward the floor.

POSITION 7: Raise the body up and place the palms on the thighs, fingers pointing forward, elbows bent. Arch the back, expand the chest, extend the neck, and allow the head to tip back slightly. Look up.

POSITION 8: Bring the head back to center, grasp the left leg behind the knee with both hands, and raise it up. Bring the abdomen toward the thigh.

POSITION 9: Lift the head, arch the back, bring the shoulders back, and look up. Bring the head back to center and release the leg.

POSITION 10: Stretch out the arms, lock the thumbs, look at the hands, and slowly fold forward from the hips. Allowing the abdomen to come toward the thighs, relax the head and the arms.

POSITION 11: Lock the thumbs, stretch the arms out, look at the hands, and slowly come up to a seated position. Continue to raise the arms up toward the ceiling. Look up.

POSITION 12: Slowly lower the arms down in front and bring the palms together at the heart center.

Relax the arms and be still for a moment, feeling the benefits of the sun salutation. It can be repeated up to three times.

SUN SALUTATION: STANDING VERSION WITH CHAIR

Stand facing the seat of a straight-backed chair. Be sure that the chair is placed so its back is against the wall for steadiness.

POSITION 1: Stand erect, feet together but not touching. Bring the palms together in front of the heart center.

POSITION 2: Lock the thumbs. Stretch the arms out from the heart center. Follow the hands as you slowly raise the arms up beside the head. Stretch up all the way from the feet to the tips of the fingers. Look up at the hands.

POSITION 3: Keeping the arms alongside the head, look at the hands and slowly fold forward from the hips, keeping the knees slightly bent. Place both hands on the seat of the chair and allow the head to relax.

POSITION 4: Stretch the left foot back, placing it on the floor a few feet behind you. Keep the left leg straight and the right knee bent. Look up.

POSITION 5: Keeping both hands on the chair and the right knee bent, lower the left knee to the floor. Arch the back. Look up and back.

POSITION 6: Bring the right leg back to meet the left. The feet are together with both knees on the floor. Pushing with the hands, straighten the legs. Look toward the feet. Stretch the heels toward the floor.

POSITION 7: Leaving the legs and arms in place, look up.

POSITION 8: Bring the left foot forward, bending the knee. The right leg remains stretched back with the foot on the floor. Look up.

POSITION 9: Lower the right knee to the floor. Look up and arch back.

POSITION 10: Keeping the hands on the chair, straighten both legs as the right leg comes forward to meet the left. Allow the head, neck, and shoulders to relax downward toward the floor.

POSITION 11: Lock the thumbs. Stretch the arms out, looking at the hands. Raise the arms up toward the ceiling as you straighten the knees and come to a standing position. Look up.

POSITION 12: Slowly allow the arms to come down in front. Bring the palms together at the heart center. Relax.

Stand quietly for a moment with your hands at the heart center and be conscious of the heartbeat and the breath. When they return to normal, relax the arms, sit down in the chair, and relax.

It can be repeated up to three times.

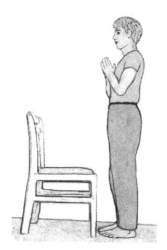

(1 and 12)

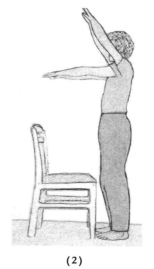

(2)

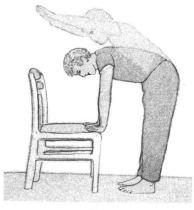

(3)

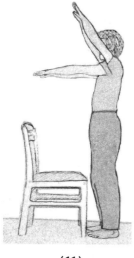

(11)

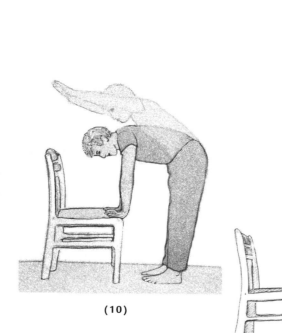

(10)

(9)

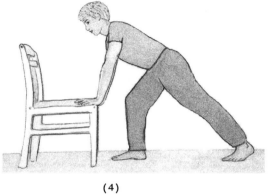

(4)

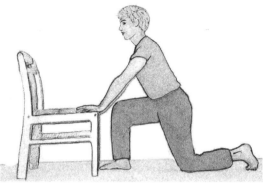

(5)

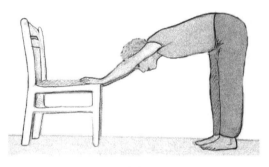

(6)

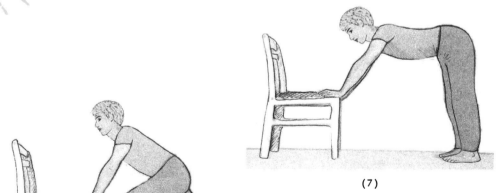

(7)

(8)

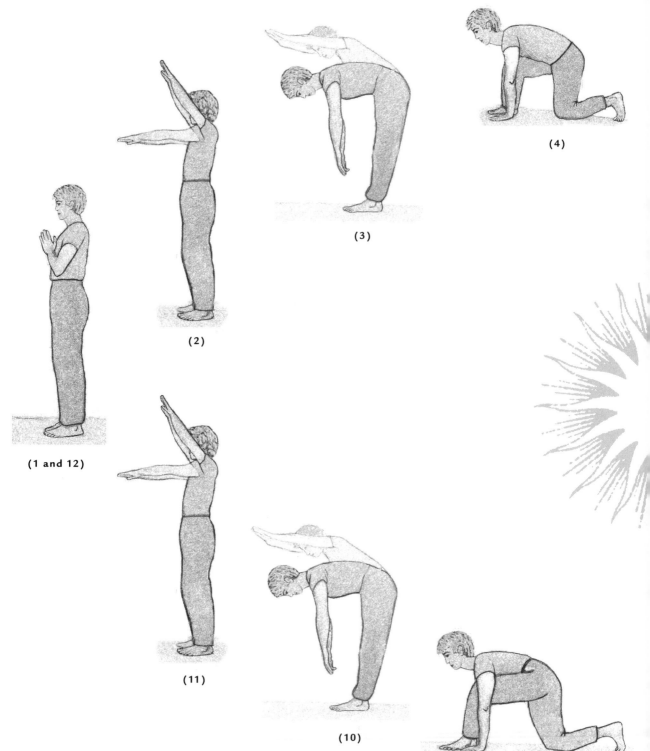

(1 and 12)

(2)

(3)

(4)

(11)

(10)

(9)

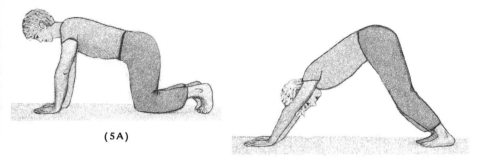

(5A)

(5)

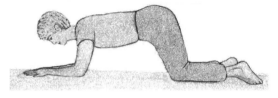

(6)

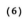

(7)

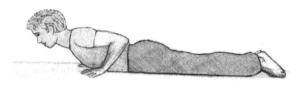

(8A)

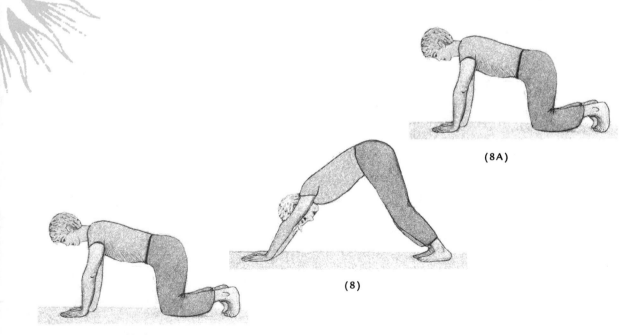

(8)

(9A)

SUN SALUTATION: STANDING VERSION

POSITION 1: Stand erect with your feet together but not touching. Bring the palms together in front of the heart center.

POSITION 2: Lock the thumbs. Stretch the arms out from the heart center. Watch the hands as you slowly raise the arms up beside the ears. Looking up at the hands, stretch up all the way from the feet to the tips of the fingers.

POSITION 3: Keeping the arms alongside the head, look at your hands and slowly fold forward from the hips, keeping the knees slightly bent. Allow the arms and head to relax toward the floor.

IMPORTANT: Practice positions 1 to 3 for a few days until the blood pressure becomes accustomed to the head moving up and down. When that feels comfortable, move on to position 4.

POSITION 4: Bend the knees deeply and place your palms alongside the outside of the feet. Stretch the left leg back, placing the left foot and knee on the floor. Leave the right knee on the floor between the hands and the right knee close to the chest. Arch the back. Look up and back.

POSITION 5A: Bring your right foot back and place your right knee on the floor beside the left knee. Both hands are on the floor (on all fours). Look up and back. (You may skip position 5.)

POSITION 5: Raise the buttocks up so that your body now forms a triangle. The hands and feet are on the floor. Stretch the heels toward the floor and look back at the feet.

POSITION 6: Slowly lower the knees to the floor and slide forward, lowering your chest and chin to the floor. Leave the pelvis slightly raised or, if more comfortable, just lower your body flat on the floor.

POSITION 7: Lower the pelvis to the floor. Have the palms on the floor beneath the shoulders, elbows close to the body and pointing upward. Gently stretch upward with the head, neck, and chest. Keep the elbows slightly bent and in toward the body. Do not push up with the hands.

We now repeat the poses going back in the opposite direction.

POSITION 8A: Pressing down with your hands and feet, lift back to the knees on all fours. (You may skip position 8.)

POSITION 8: Press down on your hands and feet to lift your buttocks and form a triangle.

POSITION 9A: Lower the buttocks. Lower the knees to the floor (all fours).

POSITION 9: Bring the left foot forward between the hands so that the left knee comes close to the chest. Look up. If this is difficult, grasp the left ankle with the left hand and bring it forward. The right leg remains with the knee on the floor.

POSITION 10: Bring the right foot forward to meet the left, bending the knees as in a squat. Allow the hands to come off the floor as your legs straighten. Keeping the knees slightly bent, allow the head, neck, and shoulders to relax downward toward the floor.

POSITION 11: With the arms still down, lock the thumbs and look out at the hands. Stretch the arms out and level with the ears. Slowly come up to a standing position. Raise the arms up toward the ceiling. Look up.

POSITION 12: Slowly bring the arms down in front and bring the palms together at the heart center.

Stand very still with the palms at the heart center. Observe the heartbeat. Observe the breath. How long do they take to return to normal? Did you strain in the poses? Is there room to stretch more?

Relax with your arms at the sides.

As you feel more comfortable with the series it can be repeated two or up to three times.

Eye Movements

Sit with the spine erect. Remove your glasses or contact lenses. We will begin to gently stretch the muscles of the eyes in all directions without any strain. If there are any areas that feel unusually tight, go even slower through those parts. Keep the head still and centered and the face, shoulders, and neck relaxed. The only thing that moves are the eyes. The breath is steady and even.

Full Circle: Clockwise Direction

Picture the face of a clock. Open your eyes and look up to twelve o'clock. Slowly begin to move the eyes to one o'clock, two, three, four, five, six, seven, and continue. Move the eyes in a smooth, flowing clockwise direction, touching each point along the clock. If the eyes want to skip a number, especially from four to six and six to eight, breathe deeply and move them even more slowly through that area. Continue a few times around the clock. As the eyes come back around to twelve o'clock, allow them to come to center, close them, and relax. Observe how the eyes feel.

FULL CIRCLE: COUNTERCLOCKWISE DIRECTION

Picture the face of a clock. Open the eyes and look up to twelve o'clock. Slowly begin to move the eyes to eleven o'clock, ten, nine, eight, seven, six, five, and continue. Move the eyes in a smooth, flowing counterclockwise direction, touching each point along the clock. If the eyes want to skip a number, especially from eight to six and six to four, breathe deeply and move them even slower through that area. Continue a few times around the clock. As the eyes come back around to twelve o'clock, allow them to come to center. Close and relax the eyes. Observe how your eyes feel.

Notice if you feel any difference between the clockwise and counterclockwise directions.

"COMPASSION

FOR MYSELF IS

THE MOST

POWERFUL

HEALER OF THEM

ALL."

—*Theodore Isaac Rubin*

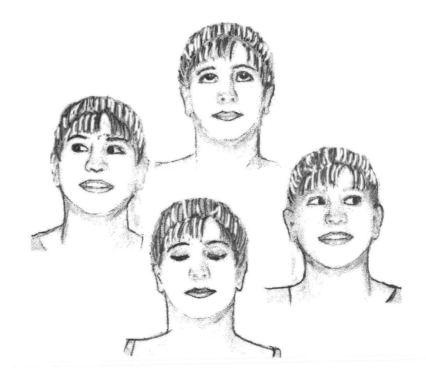

CHAPTER 7

Eating for Wholeness

TAKEN AS A PRISONER OF WAR and then isolated from his fellow inmates, Timothy was expected to survive on only a glass of water and one slice of bread each day. Although his body was being starved, it was his soul that was withering away. When he received the meager ration, all he could imagine was the satisfaction of sharing it with others in communion. Timothy envisioned cutting his one small piece of bread into four pieces. Clandestinely, he figured out a way he could give all but one of the minuscule pieces of bread to three of his fellow prisoners at exercise time each day.

To even think that others might be taking part in the same eating ritual was warm and comforting to his hungry heart. With each subsequent delivery, the risk was greater. After his successes, he would return to his cell with a sense of deep gratitude. Sitting very still, Timothy would spend a moment in silent prayer. Slowly and consciously he would eat the quarter piece of bread as if it was a great feast that he was sharing with his three "guests" and entire family. He could almost "touch" them seated with him at a grand table. Savoring each morsel, his heart and soul received more nourishment than his body.

> "ONE CANNOT LIVE BY BREAD ALONE, BUT BY EVERY WORD OF GOD."
>
> —*Old Testament*

On his liberation from prison, he was thin and frail, yet charged with vigor and health. Instead of bitterness that some felt, he was filled with the spirit of thankfulness and communion.

Ahimsa, or nonharming, is the basis for the yogic diet—in *what* we eat and *how* we eat—to do as little harm as possible.

I was talking about this concept of nonharming to one of my groups of heart patients. Many blank stares filled the faces. They diligently ate a diet low in fat and filled with nourishing vegetables, grains, and fruits, thinking only of the benefits of clearing out their arteries. They didn't realize the many other benefits that were taking place.

Finally, after spending some time talking about ahimsa, a gentle soul with the title of doctor raised his finger up just slightly. "Do you have a question or comment?" I asked hopefully.

"I have been eating a vegetarian diet now for over a year, I never thought about nonharming. Now that I reflect on it, do you think that could be the reason that butterflies land on me now?" My eyes welled up with tears and I gently said, "That could be the reason."

True ahimsa is when we have the strength and ability to do harm but instead, make the decision to do no harm, to experience a sacredness for all life.

I was sitting at a lunch counter, a young boy next to me. Both of us were enjoying burgers. Mine was a veggie burger and his was a beef burger. He eyed my sandwich with question. What was the difference? The same bun, the same ketchup, tomato, lettuce, yet something was different.

"What is that?" he finally mustered the courage to ask.

"A veggie burger," I answered, knowing exactly what he was asking.

"Why do you eat that?"

"Because I don't want to kill animals to live."

He went into deep thought and came back with this profound insight: "All the animals must love you very much." Words of wisdom from the petite kingdom!

Debra Kesten, a nutritionist and the author of *Feeding the Body, Nourishing the Soul* and a new book, *The Healing Secrets of Food,* tells how food is used as a spiritual bond in most of our cultures.

To choose and prepare food consciously gives us its life-giving properties. The Jews practice prayerful, nonviolent killing in their kosher laws. The Jains will not eat anything—even from a tree or vine—that does not willingly *fall* to the earth. Native Americans speak to the soul of the animal before the killing and promise to waste nothing. The holy Koran teaches us to kill a *larger* animal to feed a sizable gathering rather than having a small animal for each person, thereby taking only one life instead of many.

Animals and all other beings can tell when you are living with this intent of nonharming. Even as we prepare our food do it with this attitude. Whatever you choose to eat, do it with nonviolence in mind and heart.

Kesten tells a heartfelt story from the Jewish tradition where the killing of the animal is a sacred event.

A great rabbi who presided over the killing of animals for food died and was succeeded by a gentle young rabbi. The premier act of the new rabbi was watched by many eyes.

"How did he do?" others asked the onlookers.

"Oh, fine," was the nonchalant reply.

"Well," persisted the not quite satisfied group, "did he do everything right?"

"Yes."

"Didn't he recite the prayers?"

"He did."

"Didn't he sharpen the knife?"

"He did."

"Didn't he moisten the blade?"

"He did."

"What was wrong then?"

"Well," one man explained, hesitantly, "our old rabbi . . . It is just that when the old rabbi moistened the knife, he did it with his tears."

In general, we are becoming more conscious of what our food *contains,* but as yet many of us are still unaware of how we are otherwise affected by it. We know our bodies need certain nutrients to maintain their health.

Medical research is now correlating a high-fiber, lowfat diet with the prevention and even the reversal of heart disease and cancer. Many of us are becoming aware that we have too much fat, sugar, and salt in our diets. To most of us, food is more than a combination of proteins, carbohydrates, fats, vitamins, and minerals that our bodies need to be healthy. A good way to determine if something is nourishing to the body is to ascertain how close it is to its natural state; or read the labels and check the ingredients. If there are words on the label that you do not understand or cannot pronounce, *do not eat the food.* Nutritious foods are simple and nothing needs to be added or enhanced. It is better not to have to guess what you are eating or what it will do to your body.

The awareness that we have adopted about lowfat foods is sometimes ignored because we are also feeding our emotional bodies. When we do not feel nourished, we comfort ourselves by overeating and snacking on "treats" with empty calories that are high in fat. With our busy lives, we tend to eat large quantities irregularly and with much too little consciousness. Looking at our diets (not *a diet,* but the way we eat), we need to ask: Are we being nourished on physical, mental, and emotional levels?

An experiment was done with a group of people attending a seminar. Each person was asked what special foods they would like to have for lunch. As much as possible, all their culinary wishes were fulfilled in abundance.

After the full and satisfying lunch, the group was randomly divided in half and taken to two separate rooms. Both rooms were lavishly supplied with all kinds of treats—chips, pretzels, candies, chocolates, soft drinks, juices—a literal childhood fantasy. As they were seated around the table, Group One was addressed by an entertaining and motivating speaker about a topic relevant to their lives. Group Two had the misfortune to be addressed by an extremely boring speaker about a topic in which they had little or no interest. After the talks, the quantity of the food supplied was evaluated.

Group One had barely touched the food or the beverages. The lunch had physically fed them to a point of satiation. The interesting lecture had satiated their minds.

Group Two had eaten all the snacks and some even had to be refilled. They had also been physically well fed. The difference was when it came time for the mind to be fed by the lecture, it had failed to provide the needed mind food. Since there was no alternative food given to the mind, the physical food served as a substitution.

With all this information, education, and *changes* in our diet, many of us still do not feel energetic and vital. Could it be that we are not only *what* we eat, but *how* we eat?

At breakfast, the newspaper you read reports: "A two-hundred-point drop in the world stock market since yesterday, and they are predicting a drop again today." "Holiday shoppers were held hostage in a department store at gunpoint for three hours." "Rain is predicted for this weekend"— your one vacation this winter. The bond you voted against—for raising your local tax 3 percent—passed.

Enjoying your breakfast??!!

Lunch consists of dashing into a fast-food restaurant and grabbing a bite to eat, or perhaps piles of work require you to take a quick mini lunch at your desk or in the car while driving to an appointment—sandwich in one hand, cellular phone in the other.

The evening news reports how famine has affected the rural population in Africa by showing starving and emaciated babies and children. Violence has erupted in Bosnia or Israel or the Middle East. . . .

How does your favorite dish taste, the one that was lovingly prepared for your dinner??!!

Can we possibly enjoy, digest, and assimilate food when our minds are engaged elsewhere? Our mouths may chew and our throats may swallow by automatic process, yet if our mind is focused on the stock market report or shocked by violence, is it possible to digest our food fully? Is it any wonder that so many people in this country routinely use digestive aids?

Walk into any drugstore or pharmacy. We see aisles and aisles of pills and liquids to help us take care of burning stomach, heartburn, gas, constipation, and diarrhea. Add in all the headache remedies that are connected to the stomach not digesting properly. We support a large multimillion-dollar drug industry that is built around our eating improperly and not being conscious when we eat. By their own claim, these aids give us only *temporary* relief. For *permanent* relief, our eating habits must change.

Where does digestion begin? In the stomach? In the mouth? Most digestion begins with the mind.

Did you ever go to a restaurant and choose a wonderful, tantalizing dish from the menu? Your mouth waters just thinking about eating it. The digestive process has already begun. The server comes to take your order and five minutes later is back to inform you that they are out of your desired dish. How difficult is it to choose something else? Your mind, mouth, and stomach have already prepared for the first choice!

Even though your mouth never actually tasted it, your digestion had begun just by the thinking process.

To Eat or To Meet?

Have you ever had the experience of going out to lunch with a friend or to a "business luncheon"? The topic of conversation gets tense; still, you continue to eat. Only after your fork no longer has anything to lift do you notice that there is nothing left on your plate, yet you do not remember eating anything. You gingerly look under the table to see if you inadvertently dropped it there. The floor is void of food. Our bodies may have received the food, but we were not nourished.

While working on a clinical team, it seemed to be my role to remind my colleagues about being conscious at mealtimes. I would encourage them never to "eat and meet." Do only one thing at a time, I explained; "either eat *or* meet." It became common for me to be asked in advance if I would be at a certain meeting near the lunch hour. If my schedule was busy at that time, I was met with, "Oh good, without you there we can eat *while* we meet." It can be a difficult position to be the Jiminy Cricket, the conscience of the group!

The Magic Ingredient Is Love

It is small wonder that we are a society with eating disorders. We are missing the one major ingredient that McDonald's, Burger King, and even all the natural food stores combined cannot give us: *love*.

Did you ever wonder why Grandma's cookies tasted so good? She seemed to use all the same ingredients as most other cookies, ingredients that would make most of us shudder now as we recollect: white flour, white sugar, real butter, and real chocolate in generous amounts. Yet when we ate the cookies we felt happy and full of vigor. Along with the sugar and chocolate, Grandma added the most precious ingredient, *love*. As she was measuring the flour, she was feeling, *Oh, my sweet grandchild; he loves these cookies*. With each chocolate chip, *These cookies will make him strong and healthy*. And the surprising thing is, they did! Even as we smelled the fragrance from the front steps, our stomachs gurgled and our hearts leapt with joy. You may occasionally smell something that reminds you of

Grandma's cookies and it may trigger a warm feeling of *love* in your stomach and heart.

The opposite of this can also be true. Can you remember a time when you felt sick after you ate a certain kind of food? It might have been too many donuts or a crab cake you were not quite sure was fresh. Your senses were telling you, *It does not smell good; it does not look good.* But ignoring them all, you ate it anyway. Perhaps after getting sick you were unable to eat that food for weeks or months. Even now, the thought of it might make you feel queasy.

Some years back I had an experience with dried apples. Packing the apples in plastic bags for my work in the health food store, I would nibble without thinking. After some time, I began to feel very thirsty. I drank one and then another glass of cool fresh water. I went back to my bagging and nibbling, having no thought of what I had done. After a while, my abdomen started to swell like a nine-month pregnancy sped up to thirty minutes. Unfortunately, I did not have the blessing of a fast birth. Literally for days I was tasting and emitting apple gas. It took a long time to get the expanded apples out of my system. To this day, some thirty years later, I am still unable to eat a dried apple.

When food is prepared with anger we experience the opposite effect of making and serving food with love. Next time you go into a restaurant you might want to peek in the kitchen and see what kind of mood the chef is in. Is the person who waits on your table kind and cheerful? All of these vibrations will affect the food and in turn your body, mind, and emotions. There was a restaurant in the Los Angeles area that checked the staff's emotional health as well as their physical health at the beginning of each workday. Anyone who was emotionally or physically out of kilter for service was sent home for a day's rest with pay.

A friend of mine with a busy schedule teaching Yoga was late for his next class that was a one-hour drive away. As he realized that he was not going to be able to eat dinner before his next class, as if on cue, one of his students presented him with a beautifully wrapped box of homemade cookies. He was not only pleased at the gift, but also thankful for the timing. While driving to the next class, he munched on the homemade cookies. After the last class, the remainder of the cookies fueled his way home.

When he arrived home his wife greeted him with a hug and he immediately started yelling at her. The yelling accelerated into a full-blown argument, which culminated with him sleeping on the couch. The next morning, the air was brighter and lighter, and the couple talked of the night before. "What happened?" They tried to figure it out. "All we did was greet each other and then the fight started." That had never happened before in their relationship. They both embraced, shrugged it off, and went about their day.

One week later, back at the same class with the cookie baker, my friend thanked her for the delicious cookies. "Did you really like them?" she asked hesitantly.

"Yes, they tasted great!"

Relieved, she said, "I was so afraid they weren't good. While I was making them, I had a huge screaming fight with my husband. Even as the cookies were baking in the oven, we were fighting. I tried to put good vibrations in them as I was putting them in the box."

So, my friend thought, *that is the answer to the puzzle.* Perhaps if she had not put in the good vibration at the end, the fight he had with his wife could have continued through the next few days.

Conscious Preparation

Preparing and serving a meal can be an act of love. It can even be a worship service.

When we are in love or cooking for someone special, each step is important to the whole. Planning and choosing the right veggies, nuts, and grains, the balanced combinations, and then cooking the ingredients to perfection are all necessary aspects for the outcome of a great meal. Every ingredient has its part in making the dish delicious and nutritious.

Isn't it interesting that different cooks can use the same recipe but the taste of the dish will be very different? The way the food is cut, the skill and concentration of the cook are all unseen ingredients.

When I lived at the ashram, we could always tell by the taste of the food when the cook was in love. It was especially delicious!

Three Aspects of Nature

According to Yoga, all of nature, including food, reflects a predominance of one of three attributes. These attributes are called the three *gunas:*

sattwa, balance; *rajas,* overactivity; and *tamas,* inertia. The world and every-thing in it constantly moves between these three states. I like to think of them like a seesaw. There's overactivity on one side, inertia on the other, and when both are equal there is balance.

Sunrise and sunset are observed by many traditions as auspicious times for prayer and meditation, a time of equanimity. During the day *(rajas),* the light is strong; we are outward and active. At night *(tamas),* the light is withdrawn; we become more indrawn and quiet. At the moment when day merges into night and night merges into day, there is balance *(sattwa).* This balance of nature is what we hope to attain for our bodies and minds through our eating.

SATTWA: BALANCE

Sattwic, or balanced, food brings vitality and health to the body and peace and joy to the mind. It is food that is simple, tasty, and as close to its nat-ural form as possible. When food is natural, we eat less of it; our bodies are nurtured and satisfied, and our minds are in harmony. Balanced foods sat-isfy our need, not our greed. They allow us to stop when we are physically satisfied without coaxing us, "Oh, take just one more piece because it tastes so good." Do you remember the famous commercial challenging us to try to eat just one potato chip, knowing how difficult it is to take just *one?* When potatoes are thinly sliced, deep-fried in oil, and then salted, they are far from their natural state. If not stopped, perhaps many could eat the whole bag. While the potato, oil, and salt are all healthful in moderation, in opulent quantities they are not balanced and can be difficult to digest.

How many apples could you eat? Could you eat one, two? Cut them up, add lots of sugar, cinnamon, and spice, and bake them into a pie. How many apples could you eat baked as apple pie?

Sattwic food has natural vitality. When food is whole and unprocessed, we chew more thoroughly, releasing digestive juices and enzymes to aid in digestion. As food breaks down in the digestive process, it is important that it is not giving off toxins, which cause an unhealthy environment to occur in our bodies. Liquefy the food (by chewing it well) before it enters the stomach and the work of digestion is half done. With fresh whole foods each nutrient is extracted and used. The remainder of the food is easily and efficiently eliminated.

To observe the life-giving qualities I am talking about, try this easy experiment:

Take an unpeeled potato and an egg still in its shell. Put them both in the back of the refrigerator and forget about them. Ten weeks later, take them out and observe. Crack the egg and smell the sulfuric aroma of decomposing animal matter. The egg, no matter what, will never grow another egg. The potato most likely has grown roots or some of it may have dehydrated or softened. Yet you can still take the potato and plant it, and it will produce other potatoes. Even in its decomposing form, it still has life-giving properties. The potato and its properties are an example of what is meant by *sattwic* food.

Some examples of *sattwic* foods are fruits, vegetables, grains, breads, beans, nuts, seeds, and that which is in its most natural form.

Sattwic not only refers to solid food but to liquids we consume. Water is an essential part of our life on this earth. Our bodies are composed mostly of water. Yet in most cases we will drink anything *but* water. We consume large quantities of coffee, tea, soft drinks, and alcoholic beverages. Many of our physical problems can be helped by drinking just *plain H_2O.*

A doctor friend of mine always reminds us that it may not be the aspirin that cures the headache or pain, but the large glass of water you drink with it.

A dog and a man were weighed and each put on a walking treadmill for one hour. At the end of the hour they were given as much water to drink as they wanted, then both were weighed again. The dog drank enough water to bring his weight back to where it started; the man only half. Somewhere along the way we have lost contact with what the body needs and when.

Balanced eating produces a healthy body and a calm, efficient mind.

RAJAS: STIMULATION

Rajasic food is overstimulating food that causes restlessness, disease, and agitation in the body and mind.

It affects the peaceful qualities of body and mind. Food and drinks, like meat and alcohol, first have a stimulating effect and then cause you to be lethargic. After a few alcoholic drinks, you may be the life of the party.

Then the stimulation wears off and you can hardly keep your head up.

We also use food for energy or heat according to the climate we live in. In a hot climate, we tend to move more slowly. If we move too quickly or play vigorous sports, we get overheated and exhausted. Also, with the hot climate, food tends to spoil easier. Adding a bit of spice to the food acts to preserve its freshness and helps overcome heat-causing exhaustion. The spices help us to perspire, which aids the cooling system of our bodies. Transpose that same food into a cooler climate and it can cause dehydration and overstimulation.

When we overuse spices in a cold climate, instead of their giving us a little zip to get us going, they accelerate us into high speed, then cause indigestion and tempers to flare by causing too much heat or fire in the system. In moderate quantities spices can be used to stimulate the digestion and tickle the palate.

If we use too much overstimulating food it can encourage the passions to rise and the mind to become very restless. As a monk for many years, I was well aware of these effects and was interested to learn that this way of eating is observed in other religious orders as well.

While visiting in Montreal, I was invited to the inner sanctum of a Carmelite convent. Since the Carmelites are a contemplative order, mostly in silence, it was unusual for a guest to be admitted. During my audience with the Mother Superior, she asked me about my natural foods diet. Could I perhaps share some recipes with them? Surprised, I asked if they also ate vegetarian food. "Yes," she quietly told me. "Most of the contemplative orders eat this way. The mind seems to stay calmer, more available for contemplation and prayer."

I was happy to know that these findings stretched across any religious front. When the experience is the same, that supports the action.

Rajasic food can be as commonplace as coffee or black tea, which overstimulates the body and mind. Have you experienced your heart racing from too much coffee? Many of us drank coffee to keep awake at some time in our lives, perhaps when we were students or had a long night's drive ahead.

A man I once knew was very kind and friendly until he had a cup of black tea. After that, he became sarcastic and cutting in his comments to us. When we tried to tell him how his manner affected others, he would become very defensive and tell us we were ridiculous. It is sometimes difficult to know how our own actions and speech can affect others and harder to believe that a simple cup of tea can stir us to that action.

Rajasic food causes restlessness in the body and in the mind.

TAMAS: INERTIA

Tamasic food is any food that takes—instead of gives—energy from body and mind.

Food that is old or cold, overly fermented, moldy, or overcooked is considered *tamasic*. Dead and decaying food cannot give us vitality and life. The pot of soup you made last week that you just found in the back of the refrigerator probably has very little vitality left in it. Better to throw it away or compost it than to eat food without energy.

On its own, food will break down even in the refrigerator. The warmth of a 98.6-degree body allows the breakdown and fermentation of food to happen more rapidly.

Some "food" is so absent of any nutritional value, it actually depletes our energy. A friend of mine is doing an experiment with a packaged cake that has almost no nutritional value and has—to many discriminating palates—little taste as well. She bought a package of these cakes ten months before I started writing this chapter and she set one on the kitchen counter. After ten months sitting out in the open air it has not in any way started to decompose or rot. It does change texture with the weather. In moist weather it gets spongy, and in dry weather it's harder. Every time I go there I ask about the status of the cake. Is this something we want to eat to nourish our bodies and minds? Yet millions are consumed each year.

Overeating is a form of numbing ourselves. To what? Our lives, family, friends? Holidays in the United States have become a time of feasting. Cooking huge quantities of food, we eat as much as we possibly can. Waiting a few hours, we eat some more. Drowsiness comes, then sleep, and then more eating. The next day we hear cries, "Oh, I feel awful! I ate too much at Thanksgiving." At the next celebration, instead of overindulging, take the time to eat consciously. Enjoy each bite of food and be truly grateful for the abundance you have.

Many cultures will not permit food to be reheated or cooked again. They understand that food loses energy, becomes *tamasic*. What about all those leftover turkey parts after Thanksgiving? Think about reheated foods lacking energy when you see burgers piled up under hot lights. How much vitality is left after the food has sat for hours or even days? Is there still enough energy left in it to get you through the afternoon's activities?

I was teaching at a Yoga conference in Italy—one of my favorite countries for eating because of all the fresh pasta and vegetables, especially leafy green ones. After a few days, all the waiters knew that I loved the pasta and fresh vegetables the best, better than the other dishes. Instead of the regular side dish of pasta, they would bring me a full-size helping. The Italians consider it very important that the pasta be freshly made, cooked, and piping hot for full rich taste and nutrition.

One night as I was patiently waiting for the pasta to arrive, I remembered that I had left something very valuable in my room. Just as I was about to go and put it away, the pasta arrived. It was glorious, freshly prepared and made to order. "Please," I said to my table neighbor, "do not let them take my pasta. I'll be back in less than a minute." With jackrabbit speed I went up to my room, hid the treasure, and was back at the table in less than one minute. But, alas, it was too late. The luscious plate of pasta was gone. "There was not a thing I could do," said my guard. "The waiter insisted that you were to have it fresh and steaming hot. They are making you some more right now." With patience waning and appetite soaring, I anticipated the already boiling pasta. It was as good as expected!

In Yoga, we speak about toxins in the body and mind. It is a simple word that explains a buildup of unwanted chemicals and substances the body is unable to use as fuel. This can be seen as lactic acid, uric acid, or an overabundance of fats and sugars, which manifests as general aches and pains and ultimately disease. In the mind it is perceived as a feeling of fatigue, restlessness, grumpiness, or irritability. When we eat foods that do not get fully digested or assimilated, toxins take up residence in the body and mind.

Did you ever receive a gift that you didn't like but could not return or throw away? After all, it *was* given with love. Not knowing what to do with it, you put it on the top shelf of a closet. Our bodies also have "closets," places where we store what we eat that the body cannot use. The arteries are nice, open pipes where we store unusable fats and cholesterol. Our joints have crevices that are perfect for storing "toxins." When enough time has passed, the arteries may clog and the joints may ache and swell. When eating lighter, more wholesome foods that the body can digest and assimilate, there is no need to store the excesses in the body's "closets."

Tamasic food is food that takes rather than gives nourishment.

A Breath and a Prayer

The three qualities of nature apply not only to the foods themselves but also to the way in which we eat them.

Most foods can be enriched by imparting a blessing or a prayer of thankfulness before eating. This is a custom that has spanned thousands of years through feasts and famines. Taking a moment of silence can transform the food and taste, making it truly ambrosia for the soul.

Most traditions teach us to pray, chant, or take a minute of silence to prepare our bodies for the nourishment it is about to receive. While traveling in India, I met many holy people. Some lived alone by sacred rivers, in forests, or on mountains; some lived in ashrams. One teacher gave me a great lesson by his humble actions. His example stays firmly in my mind and heart.

We were already on the bus leaving Rishikesh, the "City of Saints," when a group of children came up to the bus begging for food. This was a scene we grew accustomed to as we hardened our hearts to the poverty in this land of dichotomies.

They appeared well fed (by Indian standards) to our now-jaded eyes. The bus began to move on. Then I saw *him* standing quietly in the back of the crowd of yelling children. His eyes sparkled like diamonds. His hands were together at his heart in a gesture of greeting: *Namaste.* In the stillness of his gaze, he was asking for food. When my eyes touched his, I knew I must offer him food to feed his physical body. "Please stop," I instructed the bus driver. Searching my supplies for our long trip, I found a small bunch of ripe bananas. Walking to the open door and reaching past the sea of outstretched arms, I handed this humble, yet mighty man my modest offering. The doors of the bus closed and started to move away. I watched as—with great dignity—he began slowly to peel the banana. His hunger was apparent, yet he paused. With palms together in a blessing, he looked up at me with deep pools of radiant light and blessed me for the simple gift of food. The ripe bananas appeared like stamens in the center of the radiant flower formed by his hands. By taking this moment in time before eating, the essence of the food was nourishing him—and also blessing me for giving—before the actual physical food was taken. The memory of this lesson still feeds me.

As we sit down to our daily meals, take a moment to appreciate the food—from the one who planted it in the soil, to the rain that nourished it, the harvesting, the purchase, the preparation, and the serving. With your plate of food in front of you, take in a deep breath, slow yourself down, and be aware of the intricate complexity of your body turning the food into hair and skin, bone and muscle, thoughts and love. Appreciate all the energy it will take our bodies to digest and assimilate it. You may have a certain special prayer or poem that you have learned to say before meals. If not, you can be silent or let your heart speak.

When I shared a meal with friends, their children would spend a few minutes singing before meals, "For health and strength and daily food, we give thee thanks, O Lord." It was sweet and simple and fun; we would all join in together.

One blessing I often use to acknowledge food is from the yogic tradition:

Beloved Mother Nature, you are here on our table as our food. You are endlessly bountiful, benefactress of all. Please grant us health and strength, wisdom and dispassion to find permanent peace and joy. May the entire universe be ever filled with peace and joy, love and light.

Can prayer and meditating before meals actually help us with our digestion? As modern science studies the effects of these ancient practices, we find agreement on the benefits.

A recent study was done to compare the effects of meditating for five minutes before a meal to doing difficult math problems for five minutes before a meal. It was found that the production of alpha-amylase—an enzyme found in the saliva that helps digest carbohydrate-rich food, such as pasta, cereal, and bread—*increased* with meditation and *decreased* by 22 percent with math problems.

Taking even one minute to be still and quiet allows the body to be healthier and the mind to be more at peace. It allows a transitional time between activity and eating.

Engage All the Senses

The sense of taste is the main sense used when we think of food. Yet we eat more fully when we engage as many of the senses as possible.

There is a food meditation that I do at some of my seminars. Three or four different foods are given to each person. (This is described at the end of the chapter.) They are guided through the different senses with each of the foods, the last being taste. How amazed they are to find that the ears hear the food sounds as well as the eyes seeing, the nose smelling, and the tongue and mouth tasting them.

In many cultures the presentation or visual aspect of food is of utmost importance. If the eyes are pleased the anticipation of taste is heightened. Appreciating the aroma of a sumptuous meal encourages the sense of smell to participate. Some love to hear themselves crunch and crackle while eating popcorn or chips; it adds to the full experience.

The sense that is least used for eating is the sense of touch. After childhood, we touch our food very seldom. Even during childhood, we are scolded for touching or playing with our food. Perhaps, as adults, we are *permitted* to use our hands for what are called finger foods—sandwiches, chips, and so on. As mature adults, it is unthinkable to eat mashed potatoes or salad with our hands!

The sense of touch is attributed to our hearts. This loving energy comes from the heart down the arms and into the hands. We can clearly experience that when we are embraced by someone with love.

Did you ever notice the difference in taste between food chopped by hand and food chopped by a food processor? The food chopped by hand allows the heart energy to flow into the food and keep the vital energy alive. Food chopped by a food processor misses that necessary ingredient. Salad bars are a great example of this. All the vegetables look so good and yet they often have little taste. The vital energy is missing.

The sense of taste and the action of speech are the duties of one organ. The tongue gets lots of exercise during our waking hours. We ask it to mix our food over, under, and around the teeth and mouth. We also ask it to form our words and speech. The trouble comes when we give it two jobs to do at one time. Did you ever think your tongue to be a piece of food and bite it by mistake? Engaging in conversation while eating compromises both of the tongue's functions. It can neither speak nor mix well.

Try having an entire meal or part of it in silence, without talking, reading, or watching TV. This gives us a chance to concentrate on eating. It brings awareness to the sensuous aspect of eating as well as enhancing the digestion.

In my travels around the world, it is interesting to observe how different cultures eat. When taking another look at the fork that we use every day as our main eating tool, I've thought that it could be taken for an unfriendly weapon. With sharp prongs, we stab our food and must be careful not to miss the mouth. In some countries, they use both a fork and knife together. Better to keep silence or have the conversation light, in this case, lest someone with a knife and fork in hand got upset: Watch out! Proper etiquette in those countries is to keep the prongs of the fork pointing downward and the knife's sharp edge directed at the user. Good manners have practical advantages.

In Asian countries, the eating utensils are softer. Two wooden sticks pick up the food; sometimes they are blunt, sometimes sharp. Spearing and/or extracting food from a common eating bowl brings instant communion at each meal. The soft, rounded, and nonthreatening spoon is the utensil of choice for feeding babies and in many places even for adults.

In India—as well as in other countries, including the Middle East—the natural eating implement is one's own hand. The hand is used for all foods, including soups. It is quite a feat to use the hand to drink soup and actually get some in your mouth. You may also use the hand to pick up the soup cup and drink. The benefit of eating with your hand is the direct contact with the food you are eating. The texture can be appreciated and the hand can monitor the temperature. This can save the tongue from getting scalded!

The tactile sense may not be socially acceptable in the West for people over three years old, yet we need to keep that sense alive. When you are eating at home, experiment with the way the taste changes when you eat using your fork and knife, wooden chopsticks, a spoon, or even your hands. Enjoy!

Fine and expensive restaurants treat us to a cornucopia of stimulation for all our senses. Upon entering, we experience soft light aglow with candles. There's the plushness of the carpet, the soft music, the stateliness of the chairs, the abundance of flowers, the sparkle of the crystal glasses, and the glistening of many silver knives, forks, and spoons. The delicate aroma wafts from all directions to tickle your digestion. Even the menu feeds you with its vivid and exotic descriptions. It can make a plain lettuce salad sound unique and exciting. By the time you are actually ready to ingest the food, you have been generously fed with beauty and graciousness.

This process can be done in your own home, transforming an ordinary meal into a special occasion. My memories of Sunday dinner as a child are of linen tablecloths, fine china and crystal, and the family joining together. Most of us today lead very busy lives and do not even take the time to cook. A time-thrifty friend of mine was asked if he cooked. He replied, "I don't know how to cook, but I am a great warmer."

One of the ways my husband and I have continued gracious dining in our home is to have the tablecloth on and the candles in place all the time. This allows even a simple bowl of oatmeal or take-out sushi to be treated as a gracious occasion. In certain parts of northern Europe, candles are lit even at breakfast.

Having some friends over for dinner one evening, I had prepared a simple dish. The table was set, candles lit, soft music playing. We gathered at the table and I went to shut off the nearby lamp. When the electric light was extinguished and only the candlelight was glowing, one of our guests let out an audible sigh, letting go of the day's thoughts and burdens. He had been fed before he even ate the physical food.

Even if you are not the type to use a tablecloth and fine dishes, allow the place where you eat to carry a peaceful vibration.

Fasting

In this day of eating disorders and skipped meals, fasting is not very well understood. In the past, fasting was considered a spiritual practice as well as a physical cleansing.

The belief of many natural health practitioners and spiritual traditions is that disease comes from undigested food that then creates toxins and problems in the body. By fasting, the fire of the appetite is increased, and the body burns up the unwanted toxins and is purged of them. The healing process is quickened.

Sri Swami Sivananda, a great master of yoga—who was himself a medical doctor—often said that disease can be avoided if you wait until the stomach is empty before filling it again. One of his favorite sayings was:

"It is better to fast than to eat fast."

Many religions use fasting to lighten the body and clear the mind. In this way we are able to feel a depth within or clearly experience the meaning of the holy prayers we recite.

In Christianity during the period of Lent, a special food or drink is eliminated from the diet so that in *that* sacrifice, the greater sacrifice of the Lord Jesus Christ can be felt.

The Moslem Ramadan prohibits the taking of food until the sun sets to increase the concentration of the daily prayer.

In Judaism, Yom Kippur is the Day of Atonement; on this day, the practice of fasting from food and even taking water is strictly observed. This most holy of days is a time of purification that follows the welcoming of the new year.

In Hinduism and Buddhism alike, it is a common practice to fast before and during holy days, on the new and full moon, and before rites of passage to purify the body, mind, and spirit.

On holidays, sabbaths, and celebrations, people come together around food and the joy of abundance. Sometimes we take in too much of the physical food and not enough of the spiritual food.

When beginning the practice of fasting, start slowly. Many great enthusiasts will begin with a long fast and find that it is an unpleasant experience. Take it slowly and as you feel comfortable, build up. Remember to drink lots of water!

Stage I of fasting could be for just a few hours. Have your regular breakfast and then instead of eating lunch, use that time to practice yoga poses or do breathing practices. If you begin to feel hungry in the afternoon, sip on some herbal tea or even vegetable juice or broth. When dinnertime comes, enjoy your meal in moderation, with renewed appreciation.

If that goes well, try Stage II. Have your regular lunch and then omit dinner. Again, use the time you would have allotted for dinner to do some yoga practices. The next morning, enjoy a regular breakfast. If you fast from after lunch (around 1:00 P.M. or 2:00 P.M.) until breakfast (around 7:00 A.M.) you will have fasted for about eighteen hours. The best part is that for most of the time you will have been asleep!

Stage III can be a fast from after lunch one day until lunch the next day. That will give you a full twenty-four hours of fasting. That is sufficient for a regular once-a-week or once-a-month healing fast. Longer ones can be added as the practice feels more comfortable.

One of the most important aspects of fasting is not to overeat at the meal following the fast. If you find you are too hungry by the time you reach the next meal, make the fasting period shorter. Drink lots of liquids to flush out the system and keep it hydrated. When you eat that break-fast meal, chew slowly so you are aware when you have had enough. It takes about twenty minutes for us to get the signal that our blood sugar level is back to normal and we do not need any more food. By then, most of us have eaten more than we need and sometimes more than we can digest! Hopefully, you will find fasting an enjoyable practice. You will certainly be able to use the time you have gained by not having to shop, prepare, eat, digest, and clean up from the meal.

PRACTICE OF FOOD MEDITATION

This is a fun way to begin to strengthen and clear all of your senses. When the senses are sharpened, they become a reflection of your inner as well as outer states and experiences.

In the beginning of the practice, choose foods that have definite visual, auditory, olfactory, and tactile sensations. After your senses are cleansed, more subtle foods can be used.

Have the following foods cut on a plate before you:
  a thick, fresh (not stale) cracker
  a freshly cut wedge of lemon
  a slice of a very ripe banana
After seeing the food, it is best to close the eyes and let the other senses take over.
Pick up the cracker.
Feel its texture. Is it smooth or rough?
Using both hands, bring the cracker to your ear. Break it in two. Notice how it sounds.
Bring it to your nose and notice if the aroma is stronger where the cracker was broken.
Place it on your lips and feel its texture.

Take a small bite and allow it to dissolve in your mouth without chewing. Notice how it dissolves part by part. Chew whatever is left and feel the sensation of swallowing solid food.

Can you feel it entering your stomach?

Sit quietly for a few moments and notice how you feel.

Next, pick up the lemon.

Feel its texture. Does it feel wet? Cool? How does the feel of the inner part compare with the rind?

Bring it up to your nose and smell the lemon. Does just smelling it make you salivate?

Now bring it up to your lips and rub it on the inside of your lower lip.

Place it in your mouth and notice which part of the tongue can taste the sourness of the lemon.

Feel the sensation of liquid moving down the throat as you swallow.

Can you feel it as it enters your stomach?

Sit quietly for a few moments and notice how you feel.

Next, pick up the banana.

Bring it up to your nose. How does it smell?

Squeeze the banana between your fingers. What does it feel like? What is the texture? Are you making an unpleasant face as you mash the banana in your hand?

Smell it once again. Does it smell stronger than the first time?

Place a small amount in your mouth and notice where the taste is recognized in your mouth.

Move it around with your tongue. Can you make it dissolve without chewing it?

Notice the texture as it moves down your throat as you swallow.

Can you feel it as it enters your stomach?

Sit quietly for a few moments and notice how you feel.

Observe how each of the foods looked, felt, smelled, sounded, and tasted completely different, how each of your senses was engaged in a different way.

After doing this meditation, you will hopefully experience everyday food and eating with a new awareness. You can even do this in a modified form at mealtimes. You may notice that you eat less and enjoy it more!

> "THE SKY IS THE
>
> DAILY BREAD OF
>
> THE EYES."
>
> —*Ralph Waldo Emerson*

CHAPTER 8

Prelude to Sleep

"THAT WE ARE NOT

MUCH SICKER AND

MUCH MADDER

THAN WE ARE IS

DUE EXCLUSIVELY

TO THAT MOST

BLESSED AND

BLESSING OF ALL

NATURAL

GRACES, SLEEP."

—*Aldous Huxley*

THE STARS IN THE FIRMAMENT are sparkling like diamonds. The sun is tucked gently under the earth. Time to move from your outward day into your inward night.

It is eleven o'clock at night. The day is finished. It has been very full. Eight hours of work with only a quick stop for lunch, dinner out with a friend, an evening class, catching up on correspondence, or getting things ready for tomorrow. Exhausted, you lie down in bed wanting to sleep. The body is ready to rest, but the mind is still whirling, tossing, and turning until finally you fall into a restless sleep.

Sometime in the middle of the night you awaken and the mind, holding the tired body captive, begins to roam wildly. You think about work, the new person who moved in next door, what you will say at the ten-minute talk you must give at the luncheon meeting, and so on. Every thought takes you further from a restful sleep. With each glance at the clock you begin to worry about how tired you will be in the morning. When the dawn finally comes you feel as though a battle has been fought rather than a night's rest.

We were all contented and slept well in our first bedroom. There we slept continuously, floating, surrounded and supported against gravity's pull by a gelatinous fluid the same temperature as our body. Our world was simple, each need administered to without our intervention. Comfort and love were our natural companions. Suddenly one day we were launched onto this foreign planet. Stunned, we fulfill an agreement most of us do not remember we made. Drawing in, we accept the earth's atmosphere deep into our lungs. Gaia does not have the same support or self-containment of your abandoned sanctuary. Here we must breathe, eat, and move in order to live. Adjusting to this somewhat hostile atmosphere is difficult at first. Perhaps that is why we cry out immediately after the first breath.

Sleep allows us to stay connected to our deeper source. As newborns, we sleep almost constantly. The more we acclimate to the physical demands of earth, our sleep lessens—twelve hours for children, then ten hours for adolescents, and eight hours for adults. In old age our sleep becomes short and sporadic as we approach the inevitable severance with the earth. We adjust our sleep as our dwindling allotment of days becomes a reality. Concluding our time here, we hoard the waking moments. On the final exhalation we return the borrowed breath and the voyage continues. All told, we have spent one third of our life on this earth in bed!

Over 50 percent of all Americans report some sort of sleep disturbance. Some have difficulty falling asleep, others staying asleep or restlessness during sleep and even nightmares. Why should this be? With a nation that has so many material benefits, we also have much stress.

All day long we gather words, sights, and sounds. Everything we do and think in a day is stored in our physical and subtle bodies. What we choose to read, watch, listen to, and eat has a large influence on how we rest.

As we enter into the sleep state at night, our physical and subtle bodies go into cleansing mode. Whatever has been ingested by any and all of the senses is brought back in its gross or subtle form at night. It is all sorted and either absorbed, eliminated, or stored. In dreams and deep sleep states we rid our bodies and minds of unnecessary by-products and release thoughts.

The process is similar to the way a cow processes her physical food. When a cow eats she takes in lots of grass and deposits it in one of several stomachs. All that has been gathered is not meant for consumption; it is

eat. But she, like us, takes it all in and later brings it back
f what is not appropriate to consume. There may be many
es among the sweet grass and they must be eliminated
otion of nutrients can take place.

d stones for us may appear physically as too much sugar
ies and mentally as fears, worries, and anxieties in the
he day's gatherings were restorative or calming will
ng they take us to process. Only after the sorting and
resting begin.

nuch food at the wrong times and in large quantities,
unable to balance the time allotted for cleansing, repair, and rejuvenation.

When the mind and body are not *both* focused on eating, digestion is
impeded. The work that should have been done at the time of eating is put
off until later and the stomach is called into overtime work, often at night.

Food for the body comes in all forms, not just physical. Develop the
awareness of how each thing affects you. Notice what kind of mental food
you give your mind before bed. Do you ever wonder why you had that
crazy dream? Where could the idea possibly have come from?

What we read has a direct influence on what we dream. We draw the
words and images deep into the mind. Sometimes we wake up feeling like
we have been involved in a war. Could it be from that war epic you read
last night? Late at night when the rest of the mind is still, we draw deep
within to our book, now reissued with us as the star. Will those books on
your night table lead you to peaceful sleep or will you be chasing that spy
all night long?

It is interesting that as children we enjoyed bedtime stories. Many
were of heroes, some of lofty goals taking us on a cloud to dreamland. I
do wonder why some prayers and lullabies have phrases that could actually scare adults, let alone children: "When the bough breaks, the cradle
will fall and down will come baby, cradle and all." "If I die before I wake,
I pray to God my soul to take." These seem like frightening thoughts to
hear before bed.

There are now many books designed to offer us a page or two of
inspiring or funny stories. If it is your choice to read before you drift off
to sleep, read a sweet bedtime tale, something that will allow you to smile
into your dreams, stories to inspire your dreams of hope and comfort.

The mind replays our day and all the exciting and stimulating news. How much do you watch TV or read the newspaper right before bed? It has become a practice in this country to have a TV in the bedroom, often just at the foot of the bed. Some are equipped with timers so we can drift into sleep with TV images dancing in our heads (instead of sugarplums). Many people use the news of the day as the last visual and auditory images before falling asleep. When I mention to some clients that perhaps watching TV news before bed could upset their sleep, they seem surprised. The violence and abuse that is projected at the foot of our bed may be next projected into our dreams. We incorporate the picture and sound into our sleep, the lullaby of adulthood.

It is estimated that TV waves continue to emit radiation for three hours or longer after the set is turned off! In our active lives computer, radio, TV, and microwaves are constantly bombarding us on many levels. We deserve the benefit of calm vibrations in the bedroom, free from these disturbing and perhaps damaging waves.

If, because of space constraints, a TV or computer is necessary in the bedroom or sleep area, have it screened off and turned away from the bed for sleeping time. Enjoy the difference it makes.

Sleep and dreams are healers, bringing physical, mental, and spiritual solace.

Drawing Inward

The way we design and utilize our bedrooms has an effect on our nights and subsequently our days. We can transform them into a joyful and peaceful life or a somewhat tumultuous one.

The bedroom helps us transition from daily activity to the stillness of night. Observe the place or room where you sleep. Is it a peaceful place, free from clutter? Are the pictures and colors conducive to drawing you inward? Is there a desk piled with work in close proximity to your bed, reminding you of how much you need to do? How are you awakened in the morning to greet the new day? Is there a phone beside your bed, leaving you vulnerable for an unsolicited call? What message does your bedroom give you about relaxation?

The subtle balance between sleeping and waking can be present in the delicacy of your decor. As *everything* affects your sleep and dreams, allow only the most serene and gentle vibrations to enter. In the rest of the house, all of our senses are engaged outward. Here we draw them inward.

Be conscious of the colors and patterns you choose. What kinds of pictures are on the wall? As even the sight is drawn inward, beauty flows from visual to tactile: the feel of soft carpet under your toes, the silky feel of clean cool sheets in the summer, the comfy warmth of flannel bed linens in winter, the neck gratefully releasing its burden to the soft, embracing pillow.

While visiting a friend in a distant city, she insisted that I spend the night, offering me her son's room. Finishing a fun day and a sumptuous dinner, dessert, and conversation, my eyes half-closed, I mechanically undressed and crawled into bed. After a long restless night, I awoke, sheet scattered, pillow missing in action. Squinting my eyes to the light of day, I saw this horrible, large pointed-toothed, reptilian monster dripping blood dancing over my head. Startled, I pulled away and at a downward glance became an intergalactic space traveler. I quickly jumped back to earth, avoiding the monster with a narrow escape. The patterns of both the poster and the sheets seemed to have directly affected the pattern of my sleep and dreams, contributing to the activity of the night.

My hostess, seeing my apparent battle fatigue, apologized for the wildness of her son's bedroom. Rubbing my eyes and stifling a yawn, I smiled, thinking of my own teenage years and how life changes. A calm environment supports a calm sleep and a calm life.

Sleep like a Queen

Have the most natural of fabrics surrounding you as you sleep. In sleep the body repairs and replenishes. It manufactures new cells, breaks down worn-out ones, and reabsorbs the nutrients. Each night when we sleep the body releases approximately one to two pints of water. Soft cotton bed-clothes and sheets absorb this excess liquid, allowing us the benefit of a drier, more comfortable rest. Natural fibers also support our affinity to all of nature, which aids the healing and repair process to our bodies and minds. Wholeness is the result.

A friend of mine indulged herself and purchased some very expensive natural fiber sheets for her bed. When her husband found out he admonished her for the extravagance. Confident of her decision, her words still echo in my head: "I may work like a dog every day, but I'm going to sleep like a queen every night!"

Darkness and Light

Have a balance of darkness and sunlight filling your bedroom. We sleep deeper and longer when there is darkness. How much more difficult it is to get up in the dark on winter mornings than on bright summer mornings.

Because of our modern way of life we are seldom in desert darkness. Away from the city lights, we gaze in wonder at the infinite roof over our heads. Streetlights impede our stargazing. Unless you are one of the desert dwellers, use a heavy curtain, shade, or blind to block out the evening streetlights. Allow darkness to become a cocoon wrapping you up for the long, deep sleep ahead. In the morning the butterfly emerges.

There is much evidence available to show that the hormone melatonin aids us in deep, restful sleep. This is a hormone naturally produced and secreted by the pineal gland when we are in darkness.

While I was leading a seminar in Italy, the students requested time after lunch for their customary siesta. Gathering after the rest, we spoke about the fading of this healthy and relaxing custom. Busy lives eliminate any unnecessary niceties, even ones bound in tradition. One student spoke up. He was a scientist, sharing evidence to justify the usefulness of the afternoon rest. It had been studied and proven that closing the eyes in darkness and actually touching sleep, for even an instant, released melatonin into the bloodstream. This liberated energy and alertness sustains us for the remainder of the day, a scientific validation for a nap. We spend millions of dollars to prove common sense!

Allow the light to stream into the bedroom during the daytime. Open the windows fully to aerate the room each day. The sunshine and air allow the staleness, odors, and unwanted thoughts and feelings to vanish. Native Americans use a webbed circle with feathers called a "dream catcher." True to their name, they hold onto bad dreams until they can be released in the morning. By aerating, all unwanted thoughts and dreams are replaced by fresh rejuvenated energy.

When I was teaching in Germany, each break would create an aerating session. Summer or winter, rain or dry would not matter. All doors and windows were flung open and deep breaths were taken. The minds and bodies were refreshed, alert, and open for the next session of class. We became like little champagne bottles with the corks popped and ready for action.

Attack!

You have left your beautiful home for an outing to the lake. The day is clear, the sun warm on your skin, the smell of jasmine in the air. The hum of bees is heard nearby as they dance in the air with their winged companions. Reaching your favorite destination, you relax. Suddenly you hear this terrible and loud buzzing noise. Could the bees have gotten that loud? You begin to feel fear. Your voice fails as you try to cry out in desperation. The noise gets louder! As you turn to run, the stable legs of moments ago are now worthless blobs of jelly. *BUZZ! BUZZ! BUZZ!* What to do? Your heart begins to pound, blood pressure rises, your eyes dart open, pupils dilate, blood rushes to the legs and arms. *RING! BUZZ! RING!* We are alerted to danger. An attack? Run for your life! *RING! BUZZ! RING!*

This fight-or-flight response of the sympathetic nervous system is caused by THE ALARM CLOCK! Although this is quite a violent reaction for a routine wake up, it is how most of us awaken each day. Some of our stress can be lessened *just* by changing the way we welcome a new day.

Observe the first thought that comes into your mind when you are shocked into waking: "Oh,——!" Fill in your own blank. Is that the word and tone you want to start off your day? Beginning the day with a curse or swearing, you must travel a long way for it to be peaceful.

We need *something* to beckon us to our jobs and responsibilities. When left to our own rhythm, we might miss the train or our first appointment of the day. Eliminating the alarm clock may not be a possibility. Adding a measure of delicacy may be just the soothing balm your nervous system needs. Change your *alarming* clock into a gentle *waking* clock.

There are so many different kinds of systems to choose from these days. A clock radio can be tuned to a station with appealing music. Be sure to adjust your waking time just before or just after the hour so that you are not hearing the news as your consciousness emerges: "A bomb exploded in—killing 25 and injuring 168 . . ." This image does not elicit a feeling of "Wow! What a wonderful day."

While visiting abroad, my husband and I stayed in a bedroom where the former sleeper was accustomed to rising early each day. The alarm clock radio initiated the alarm button the same time each day. At 4:00 A.M. on our first day in a new country, we were shocked out of our sleep to hear "A major earthquake rocks the Los Angeles area. Estimated property damage, injuries, and deaths are yet unknown." Our nervous systems were sent into fight and flight. Was anyone we knew hurt? Oh, those poor scared souls! Prayers for all. Will my flight to L.A. be okay? Prayers for all. For the rest of the day we experienced the aftershocks and residuals from the earthquake that had shaken our lives eight thousand miles away from the epicenter.

If possible, choose your own music or even a comedy cassette or CD. Did you ever hear a song first thing in the morning and even at two in the afternoon it is still going round and round in your head? Choose that song carefully so it will bring you a bright and positive outlook even in the late afternoon. Many systems start off softly, coaxing you gently out of your deep dreams. Upon awakening, as we struggle to fix our reality, the gradual rise in the volume allows us to surface slowly. Some clocks are connected to a light that gradually brightens until you are coaxed into awakening. It is as natural as the dawn through your window. With any of these gentle wake ups, we become fully conscious to a good morning. Waking up may not be any easier, but it will be much more pleasant!

Notice how differently we feel on weekends and vacation times when we awaken more gently and the natural rhythm of the body is honored. That message is accepted by the mind and our all-over ease is enhanced.

Whether remembered or not, we release emotions and live out many fantasies in our dreams. Some dreams we would like to forget and some we hold dear. Our daily sanity is sustained by our ability to release in our dreams. In deep, restful sleep, the essential link to our spiritual source is reestablished.

Wrong Number

When intruders are permitted to disturb our calmness without invitation, we are unable to feel totally safe. For many of us that intrusion can come in the form of a ringing phone. The sanctity of the bedroom is based on feeling safe. We all know the panic response of being startled awake by a ringing phone. Most calls that come at night do not present good news. Rarely do awards or checks for a million dollars come at 2:00 A.M.!

The sound of the phone has conditioned us to respond with alertness. The frequency of wrong numbers or friends in a different time zone calling with apologies can easily be prevented. Unless there are extenuating circumstances, such as ill parents, teenagers out late, or the like, have the ringer in the bedroom turned off. In my home I attempt to keep our nighttime sacred, so the phone ringer in our bedroom is turned off from 9:00 P.M. to 9:00 A.M. whether we are sleeping or not. The time of stillness allows us to open and become powerfully effective.

The Five Bodies in Sleep

Investigating sleep through the subtle bodies or *Maya Koshas* (see Chapter 3, Deep Rest, Deep Relaxation), we understand that there is much more to sleep than putting your head down on a soft pillow.

Accessing and acknowledging these five subtle aspects takes us into the deep and restful sleep we need to achieve optimum physical, emotional, and mental health.

Doing a few minutes of deep relaxation, physical poses, breathing, imagery, and meditation before bedtime assures us of a deep and peaceful rest. We can retreat back into our center and sleep like a baby.

The physical body, or *Anna Maya Kosha,* holds tension stored in the muscles, organs, and nerves. Each movement or strain we make during the day, the body tries to correct at night.

As the physical body is able to relax, it liberates the energy, or *prana,* from its cells, muscles, and organs. The physical body's relaxation is observed by its heaviness, a feeling of letting go.

Do you remember a time when you might have done a long hike, much longer than you would usually take? Or perhaps you visited a friend's country home and helped him chop the winter's wealth of wood? That night when you reclined into a supportive bed, the tiredness outweighed the call from the muscles for attention. The body's healing power spent the night trying to repair the overworked muscles. As we slept a buildup of lactic acid manifested as cramping in the foot or leg or stiffness and irritability in the morning.

When we are able to release the tension and stiffness *before* bed, the blood is better able to flow freely through the body. The heart and respiration, not heavily burdened by the cleansing process, slow to their restful pace. On awakening, we reaffirm life by deep breathing into our lungs. Exhaling, we let go of inflexibility and rigidity, which prevents us from learning and growing.

PRACTICE OF TECHNIQUES FOR A PEACEFUL SLEEP

Purification by Water

This yogic technique of purification by water is a great way to cleanse, release, and revitalize the physical body *and* calm the mind. In India, to bathe in the holy rivers while reciting prayers and mantras is considered a release from all problems and karmas.

Even if you are not near a holy river you can modify this technique and try it at home, making your bathtub sacred. Prepare a warm bath with a soothing aroma such as lavender. If you prefer a shower, use a scented shower gel. Light a few candles and play soft music. Allow your body to soak, the tensions to retreat as the water flows down the drain. The senses that have been bombarded during the day are soothed, relaxed, and moved inward. Let go of all the disturbing thoughts in the mind. You are finished with the "busyness" of life. There is nothing left for you to do but relax.

After the soothing and relaxing bath, practice a few gentle poses or asanas to further release tension from the physical body.

Physical Poses

NECK MOVEMENT

Neck and shoulder movements reestablish the flow of energy between head and heart. (For complete instructions, refer to Chapter 6, Move and Heal—Physical Poses.)

Sit comfortably in a chair or on the floor or a bed, shoulders and arms relaxed. Inhale. Exhale as you bend the head forward so that the chin comes toward the chest.

Breathe normally as you allow all the muscles in the back of the neck to relax. Allow the weight of the head to help stretch out the neck.

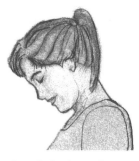

Inhale and bring the head back to the center. Exhale. Relax.

Inhale. Exhale as you slowly bring the right ear toward the right shoulder. Feel the stretch on the left

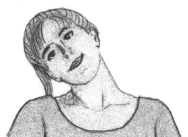

side of the neck. Keep the shoulders relaxed and the breath regular. Inhale and raise the head to center; exhale and relax. Repeat with the left side.

Exhale. Relax.

Notice if any thoughts or feelings from the day surface as you do the neck movements. Perhaps you are releasing thoughts that might have gotten lodged in the neck. You can now allow them to dissipate.

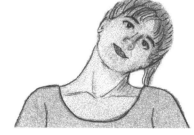

SHOULDER ROTATIONS

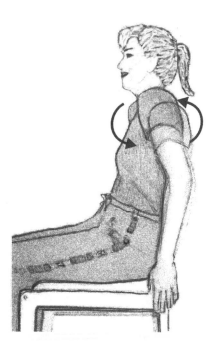

Allow the arms to dangle loosely by your sides. Slowly begin to make circular movements with the shoulders. Keep the arms and hands relaxed and at your sides so that the weight of the arms aid in the relaxation.

Keep the breath even and moving slowly through each part of the movement. Move even slower through any especially tense or sore spots, coaxing them to let go. After a few repetitions, allow the shoulders to relax. Gently shake the arms.

Repeat the same circular movements in the opposite direction.

Allow a smile to come to your face as you feel the relaxation and the energy moving freely from the heart to the head and the head to the heart, releasing any of the burdens you have been carrying all day long.

FULL FORWARD BEND

Forward bending poses are great at night to move the energy inward and upward.

Sit on the floor or bed with the legs outstretched. Have a slight bend in the knees, the toes pointing up toward the ceiling. Bring the palms together at the heart center, lock the thumbs, stretch the arms out while inhaling, stretch up toward the ceiling, and look up. Exhaling, look at the hands as you come forward over the outstretched legs, keeping the back straight and lifting from the hips. Grasp the legs wherever comfortable and allow the head, neck, and shoulders to relax while continuing to keep the chest expanded and eyes looking forward. Feel as if you are drawing the energy from the outside to the softness and protection of the inner being.

Inhale and lock the thumbs and stretch the arms out in front. Slowly come up to a seated position. Exhale as you slowly bring the arms down, palms together at the heart center. Relax completely.

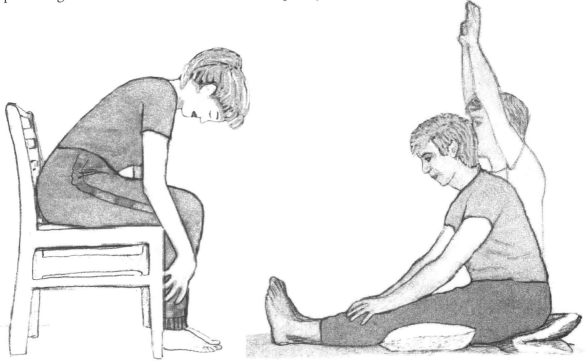

FORWARD BEND ON CHAIR   FORWARD BEND ON FLOOR

CROCODILE POSE

This can be done on the floor or in bed, right before sleep, or if you awaken in the middle of the night.

Lie on your belly, arms folded; have the head on either side. If more comfortable, have the arms at your sides. Observe the rising and falling of the abdomen as it expands and contracts with the breath.

As the belly touches the floor or bed, feel that it draws energy up from the earth. With each inhalation, feel the earth's grounding energy filling your body and mind. With the exhalation send the breath and whatever thoughts or feelings are keeping you from being peaceful back to the earth. Continue for as long as comfortable. You may find you actually fall asleep in this pose.

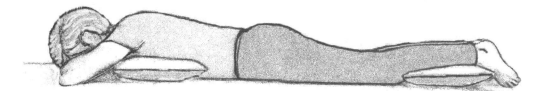

THE SEAL OF YOGA OR YOGA MUDRA

This pose is a mudra that assimilates energy and gently moves it into higher centers of consciousness away from the hubbub of our busy lives. Some of the great benefits of this pose can be felt by coming up as slowly as possible.

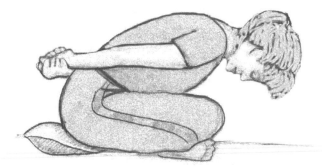

SEAL ON FLOOR

Sit in a cross-legged position or on a chair with the eyes closed. Bring the arms behind the back and grasp the right wrist. Inhale deeply and stretch up.

On the exhalation, extend the chin and with a straight back, fold your body forward over the legs. When you have come forward as much as you comfortably can, allow the body and head to relax.

As you raise back up, inhale deeply, extend the chin, and slowly allow the buoyancy of the lungs to raise the head and body up with each inhalation. With each exhalation, the body naturally comes down slightly. Continue until you are erect in a sitting position.

Keeping the eyes closed, allow your hands to come to your lap. Sit very still and feel the effect of the yogic seal. Experience the peace within.

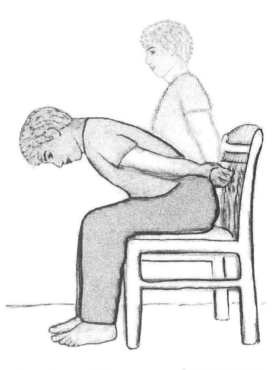

SEAL ON CHAIR

After the bathing (your water cleansing) and time of gentle stretching, allow the body and mind to continue its migration inward.

The energy body, or *Prana Maya Kosha,* is now able to move freely through and beyond the boundaries of the physical body. The more fluid the movement of the *prana,* the more relaxation occurs for the physical body. As the energy body is not needed for any elaborate movement of the body or mind, it is able to repair and revitalize cells and organs and then rest.

Observe how much energy it takes to live our lives on a regular basis. How much of that energy is wasted by unnecessary movement, eating, emotions? Do you consciously conserve your movements, actions, and speech?

Our daily practice of conscious breathing, or *pranayama,* helps us be aware of how we are using our energy. The simplest breathing practice can balance the energy that liberates the body, mind, and emotions, enhancing our ability to go into a deeper sleep. Even the smallest child, when asleep, is physically very heavy. She has let go and is abandoned to any cares of the world. When we relax our energy body, we feel a heaviness and an abandonment to the physical world.

Breathing Exercises

THREE-PART BREATH

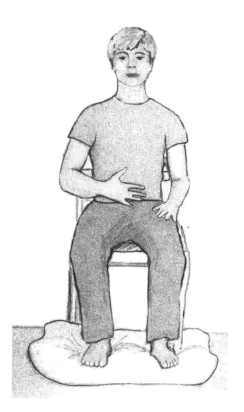

Begin to take in a deep three-part breath exhaling completely through the nose. At the end of the exhalation, contract the belly. Inhale and expand the belly, allowing the lower lungs to fill. Continue to inhale, allowing the lower chest to expand. Move the inhalation into the upper chest, allowing the collarbones to rise slightly. On the exhalation, empty the upper chest, the lower chest, the abdomen—one section flowing into the other. Inhale and continue to expand the abdomen and lower chest, the middle chest, and the upper chest so that the collarbones rise slightly. Continue breathing slowly and deeply for a few minutes.

ALTERNATE NOSTRIL BREATHING

To further relax the thinking mind and emotions, begin to do the three-part breath. Exhale fully, close off the right nostril with your thumb, and inhale slowly through the left nostril.

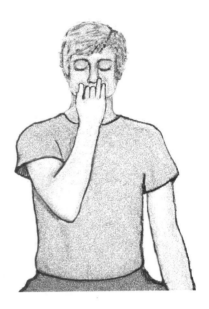

Close off the left nostril with the finger and exhale through the right nostril. Inhale through the right nostril. Close off the right nostril and exhale through the left nostril. Continue this pattern. Exhale, inhale, switch nostrils; exhale, inhale, switch. If any thoughts invade the mind, allow them to leave with the exhalation. Allow only peaceful and sleep-provoking thoughts to enter with the inhalation.

As you come around to the right nostril, end with an exhalation. Allow the hand to come to the lap and be still with the eyes closed. Observe how calm and still the breath and mind have become.

With the liberation of energy from the body, the mind *and* senses *(Mano Maya Kosha)* can use that energy to process and sort out thoughts and ideas stored in the mind. Once these thoughts and ideas are released we are able to withdraw farther from the physical realm of our consciousness.

His large size did not allow John to lie comfortably on the floor. We had to use several pillows to support his frame. After some time he was able to relax. He had a condition known as sleep apnea, where the breath stops when he is asleep. One part of his deep consciousness ventures to depths unknown to his conscious mind, causing the breath to stop. He is then suddenly awakened by another part of him. Fright is the result.

In these situations the first three stages of deep relaxation are very comforting and reassuring. By consciously directing the breath and then observing it, the mind is able to vigilantly access any hesitation of its flow.

While I was teaching, one part of my consciousness would stay focused on John. I noticed on this particular day he was very still and calm. Usually he would squirm and fidget. I sat beside him and was able to observe a steady pattern of breathing, a calmness.

When the others had left, John came up to me and asked for a minute of my time.

"I had forgotten, totally forgotten," he began. "When I was six years old, my best friend and I went into the lake to swim. We were both good swimmers. He got his leg caught on some rope that was tied to a buoy. I held my breath to go underwater to help him get loose. I couldn't hold my breath any longer and had to let go. He drowned and I told myself that I would practice holding my breath until I could hold it so long that that kind of thing would never happen again. I became the champion underwater swimmer in my town.

"As I was relaxing today, I felt my breath stop, then the memory of my friend's drowning came back to me. I had forgotten totally about why I started to hold my breath and swim underwater. By holding my breath when I slept, I was trying to punish myself for my inability to save my friend's life. My good intentions turned against me."

By John's learning how to regulate and equalize the breath the memory came up to the surface of the conscious mind after forty-six years. That night he had the first full, deep sleep he had had in years.

Draw further inward by allowing the mind to release thoughts, feelings, and regrets of what you *should* have done that day. Retrace your day from early morning and release the scenes from your mind. If your mind fixes on a particular event, examine how you could have done it differently and then let it go. You may even like to repeat an affirmation, such as: I release this day and enter into a deep sleep to repair and rejuvenate my body, mind, and spirit.

As the mind becomes simple and uncluttered there is a lightness, an upward movement away from the mundane.

We unite the body, energy, and mind by using the gentle, healing breath to soothe any thoughts and feelings from the toes, feet, lower legs, upper legs, and hips. Gently soothe the fingers, hands, arms, and shoulders. Relax. Soothe the front of the body, all the internal organs, and the back of the body. Allow the face to soften with a smile. Soothe your mind with a peaceful thought or scene, lullaby, chant, prayer, or mantra.

When the body, energy, and mind are peaceful, your sleep moves into a higher consciousness (the wisdom mind or *Vijnana Maya Kosha*). As we rest here, we are able to tap into knowledge that allows us to be creative and effective in our waking lives. Whether it is knowing how to heal ourselves, create a work of art, or master our own minds, it all comes from here. At night we are able to plug into the master computer.

Now the time has come to lie down on that soft pillow and drift into a sweet dreamless state. Giving yourself permission for a much needed rest, tuck all the remaining thoughts of yesterday, today, and tomorrow in a pillowcase and set it aside. Observe the breath as it slows and calms, drifting away from even the breath to a deep childlike sleep.

If all goes well, we may be blessed to enter the body of bliss, peace, and joy *(Ananda Maya Kosha)*. This takes us into the center of our being to the stillness, a true rest. A feeling of oneness prevails as you drift into a peaceful sleep, to sleep until you awaken with renewed vigor, vitality, and joy for a new day. We then radiate this joy to all we meet.

"ONE OF THE MOST ADVENTUROUS THINGS LEFT IS TO GO TO BED, FOR NO ONE CAN LAY A HAND ON OUR DREAMS."

—E. V. Lucas

CHAPTER 9

Great Excuses, Great Solutions

"NATURE, TIME,

AND PATIENCE

ARE THE THREE

GREAT

PHYSICANS."

—*Proverb*

I HAVE HAD THE PRIVILEGE of teaching Yoga as stress management for many years to all populations, including people with life-threatening diseases. It always amazes me how many excuses I hear for *not* doing the practices. Even though, in many cases, the practices were being prescribed after other medical treatment had failed, the impetus to do them was not there. *(I do not recommend that you do these practices instead of medical treatment unless you are doing them under the supervision of a doctor and with the aid of a fully trained Yoga teacher.)*

I often liken doing the practices to an insulin-dependent diabetic. The insulin—or, in this case, the practices—must be taken to control the disease process. To help yourself heal a physical or mental malady even more vigilance is required. If you are lucky enough to be doing these practices for prevention, I suggest that you allow them to take a strong place in your life so your goal can be achieved.

What do you need to help yourself be whole and complete? As you traveled the labyrinth, could you identify your strengths and weaknesses? Which part of your being have you focused on and which part has been neglected? Assess the different aspects:

The interaction with others and the opening of your heart

The use of the mind as an instrument, helping us to think positively, thrive, and heal

The time of rest and drawing inward to revitalize our whole being

The regulation of energy to balance our life force

The great sense of peace and assurance that comes from knowing your soul

Understanding how to strengthen the body from the inside out

To eat with an awareness of nurturing

Sleeping like a baby, awakening with joy

After going through the philosophy, chapters, and techniques, this is the time to put into practice what you have read. Were there any times in the book that you thought, *I really could use that! That really rings true for me. I wish I could control my anger like he did.* Perhaps you even underlined it or wrote it down.

The difficult part of any great program is to do it. It is great to hear how everyone else can benefit, but will it really fit into your life? Even if some reversed heart disease, cancer, chronic back pains, will it work for you?

The best thing is to try it. From my experience the more changes you can make in the beginning, the quicker you will see benefits and the better you will feel. Some of the benefits are subtle; you may not be aware of them at first. However, the advantages of *enjoying* a regular practice enhance its power greatly. Dive right in while you are inspired. Be bold.

The other way is a little more conservative and may be a bit more comfortable for you. Take on one or two of the practices that seem most likely to bring benefit. Use them diligently for at least a month (with less time it is difficult to assess the effects). After a month begin to add one of the practices or ideas that is *less* comfortable.

For example, you decided to eat a healthy diet and do some of the breathing practices for one month. You feel really well physically, mentally, and emotionally. It may be difficult for you to go out for lunch with your friends now that you eat only healthy food, but you are getting more creative and feeling more comfortable in your own conviction. What would you choose for your next practice? Perhaps take a minute out before you eat to be still.

I would suggest starting to take that moment of stillness in your own home *first.* You may feel less self-conscious and when you *feel* the benefit, you can then take it out in public. Combining that silence with deep breaths could be two practices in one!

Here are five good questions to ask yourself. Write down the answers before beginning your practice. At first, you may want to review them on a daily basis. After some time, when you feel the benefits, the answers can be reread for renewed inspiration.

1. Do I believe that a relaxing Yoga practice is an important and key component to coping with stress, preventing disease, and transforming my life?
2. What time of day will I do the practice? For how long? What will I use to inspire myself to practice regularly?
3. Which of the practices will I do and how long will I spend on each part of the practice? Will the practices be done all in one time or divided into two or more sessions?
4. Where will I create a sacred space and what will it contain?
5. How will I incorporate the practices into my everyday life?

Listed below are some of the most common excuses I have heard for not being able to *do the practices.* They are by no means the most creative. Also listed are some of my favorite solutions. You may even be able to add a few to each part yourself.

Great Excuse #1: "I Don't Have the Time."
"I'm Too Busy."

I place this as #1 because out of all the excuses I hear this comes up over 90 percent of the time. Sometimes it comes alone, sometimes wedded to other excuses.

It always amuses me to observe a dynamic and successful person shyly explaining to me why they are unable to take the time out of a busy day to concentrate on their own healing process. I would always ask the question "What else could possibly be more important than your own health and well-being?"

I tried an experiment a few years back while living at the ashram. It was then located in a very cold climate and each winter, the flu would take victim after victim. I observed that each time another casualty was taken by the *minute* virus, s/he went to bed for three days. During that time, cozied under a thick warm comforter or blanket, the "victim" read a good book and sipped herbal tea. After the three days, s/he came back to life, looking better than before. It had been a great *retreat* time.

Not enjoying sickness and wondering about prevention, I came upon an idea. Making myself a large pot of herbal tea and seizing a good book, I crawled under my fluffy comforter (interesting name: "comfort giver") for a three-day rest.

After the allotted time, I emerged refreshed and ready. The strange part was that for the rest of the flu season I seemed to be *immune,* as if I had actually *had* the disease.

This curious result encouraged me to continue the experiment next year. The same reward came again. When I took the time for my body to rest and rejuvenate *before* I became ill, the disease was averted. You may want to try the same experiment yourself!

Money, position, power, prestige, and even happiness fade in the wake of sickness. In the hospital, rich and poor, great and humble, all don the same short gown and go through the same tests and sometimes tortuous treatments. Our health is one of the most important aspects of our lives. Without it, peace and happiness are difficult.

We all have twenty-four hours in a day. How much time during your day are you willing to dedicate to keeping yourself well? Is it time to reevaluate your priorities as if your life depended on it? It does!

One day as a middle-aged man with heart disease was giving me the excuse of not having enough time to do Yoga as stress management, I gave him this puzzle:

Count up all the days that it would take for you to go to the doctor, be diagnosed, taken into the hospital, and have bypass surgery. Figure in the recovery time in the hospital and at home until you are able to return to work full time. Add up all the hours and days. That is how much time it takes to undergo and recover from bypass surgery. Divide the total by 365. Use those same hours each day for your Yoga practice and you might be able to bypass the surgery altogether!

It is interesting how we take time—maybe reluctantly—to be sick. Even with that, if we can take a pill and keep going, we will do that. Sickness is the body's way of telling us to slow down and relax.

Incorporate some simple *reminders* into your life. Some of us look at our watches twenty, fifty, or one hundred times a day. Place a small dot or string on your watch and each time you glance at it, instead of thinking about being late or in a hurry, take one deep breath. That could be one hundred deep breaths or more each day. This could be seen as a therapeutic benefit of wearing a watch—with a lifeline.

Write the word *breathe* on Post-it notes and put them in strategic spots: when you get into the car, before you answer a ringing phone, while caught in traffic, placed on hold on the phone to remind you to breathe. One of my colleagues put the word *breathe* on her screen saver and each time she uses the computer, it reminds her to breathe. Before you know it, you will be deep breathing regularly and feeling great.

Great Excuse #2: "I Don't Enjoy It. I'm Bored."

Sometimes we become very childlike when we are asked to do something for our health that is not what we would have chosen to do. Think about where the choices you have made have gotten you healthwise thus far.

Boredom comes when we expect results by a certain time. Natural healing is a slow and steady process; go deeper.

Often I will be asked if something "counts." "If I do more walking or exercise is it okay to do that instead of the Yoga poses?" Exercise is great for health, but it does not take the place of the Yoga poses. Do the exercise first and then use the poses to cool down and balance the system.

"If I quietly sit and read the newspaper, isn't that as good as meditating? That is relaxing for me. I don't like to meditate." Deep relaxation comes when both the body and mind are still and at peace.

You needn't meditate for long periods of time. At first, stop whatever you are doing for just *one moment* each hour and be still. Appreciate your heart's beat, the breath's tide, allow it to swell into a deep wave of oxygen, and slowly let go of that which you no longer need.

Most of us take ourselves *and* life too seriously. When viewed from a distance, life can be more lighthearted than when seen close-up. Step back every so often and find the humor in life's various situations. Smiling is good for physical and mental health and helps us stay lighter.

To keep yourself inspired, try to enhance your environment by playing soft, soothing music and go to group Yoga classes. Vary and add optional practices that you may particularly enjoy on a regular basis.

Great Excuse #3: "There's No Room in My House."
"I Can't Do It When I Travel."
"I Spend Ten Hours a Day at the Office."

Even a small space is big enough for practice. On occasion, when traveling and staying in a small room, I do poses, breathing, and meditation on a straight-backed chair or even on the bed. If we look for a reason to avoid doing Yoga practice, we can easily find it.

Eating a good, nutritious breakfast does not keep us fueled for the whole day. An early, midday, and evening meal are eaten for continued nourishment all day long. It is the same with Yoga practice. If we do a few minutes in the morning and then go ahead and live life just as we did before, the results are less dramatic. Doing the formal practice and then little bits throughout the day help us stay centered and calm. Don't leave the benefits behind and go off to the "real world" of worries, emotion, and tension. Incorporate some "practices" into your daily routine. Learn to use the pauses in the day as opportunities to stretch, move, breathe, and positively image. To keep that balanced feeling all day pack up a few techniques to carry along with your lunch.

Here are some great opportunities for practice "snacks" during the day no matter where we are in the world:

✘ *Sitting for long hours at your desk, computer, or car? Stuck in a traffic jam?*
   Place both hands on the wheel, table, or desk; inhale and lean forward and up as in cobra pose. Do a half spinal twist. Encourage the energy to move and flow.

   In a car or on a train, bus, or plane can be a perfect opportunity to breathe deeply, stretch, or just be quiet and listen.

× *Put on hold on the phone?*

Keep a pad and pen handy and while waiting write an uplifting word, phrase, or mantra. When the person returns, instead of being annoyed, you will feel calm and centered.

× *Waiting for your meal to come at a restaurant?*

Do arm, leg, neck, and shoulder movements. Keep the blood flowing to the stomach and digestive organs.

× *During commercials on TV?*

Do a few of the poses that easily lend themselves to chairs, i.e., forward bend to relieve tightness of the back.

× *In line at the store?*

Stand behind the counter or your cart and stretch one leg back as in half locust pose; repeat with the other leg as you move forward.

× *Doing paperwork at your desk?*

Do eye movements. Take a minute to do these once each hour and eyestrain will be a stranger.

Especially when in foreign places, the practices comfort me with a familiarity of being home. Home is where the heart and soul reside.

Great Excuse #4: "Holidays Are Difficult." "We Have Guests in Our Small House."

Holidays are traditionally a time when all our disciplines—whether with food, exercise, or practices—are diminished or even eliminated.

It takes more consciousness to keep our routine in the midst of other activities. Most friends and family will understand and even encourage us to take the time for ourselves. If they don't understand taking the time for health and healing, your good example of taking the time to do the practices might encourage them to look into their own habits. By taking this time for your own Yoga practice, you might actually inspire others.

Some years back, a busy teaching schedule in New York City allowed me little time to rest in between programs. After Saturday's workshop on

Healing the Healers, I was invited to go to a friend's house for dinner. Conscious of the events of the next day, I knew the best thing for *my* well-being was to spend the night resting. With great concern for her feelings, I gingerly approached my hostess, who had participated in the workshop.

"I feel very sorry to have to say this. I know you have been preparing and guests are invited, yet I am very tired and really need to rest tonight. I hope you can understand."

Her eyes welled with tears. Seeing her tears, I was ready to say, "Okay, let's go!" Then she spoke: "Hearing you say this teaches me more about Healing the Healer than the whole day's workshop. To really see that you practice what you teach means so much to me. It is a great lesson. Thank you. Have a great rest. See you in the morning." We often teach more by what we do than what we say.

Great Excuse #5: "I'm Too Tired or Stressed Out to Do Yoga."

This is always a funny one to me—to be too tired to do that which relieves stress. Why are you so tired? Is it because you are doing too much in your life? If that is the case, plan to do less in a day. Make your daily goals reasonable. Do less and feel less stress.

My father-in-law, Ron Gross, had some problems with his heart so he has been doing the heart disease reversal program. He was not interested in getting sicker so he took up Yoga to help him improve his health. When he puts his mind to something, his goal is accomplished. He is totally faithful to his Yoga practice. Visiting one of the residential heart retreats, he spoke to a participant, another busy businessman. The man was saying that he didn't have time in the morning to do the one hour of Yoga practice we recommend for the reversal of heart disease. Ron smiled, knowing he had thought the same way one year before.

"Look," said Ron, "when you get to your office in the morning, has your secretary finished what you gave her the night before?"

"No," replied the other man.

"Well, then, come in at 10:00 A.M. instead of 9:00 A.M. Use the hour for your practice, and, by then, the work will be ready for you."

It sounded like good advice to me. Make Yoga a priority in your life.

Are you tired because you are not exercising enough? The blood and muscles need movement. Movement is life. Do the physical stretches and poses; they will rejuvenate you. Add some walking to your daily routine. Park the car a few blocks away from your work and walk the rest of the way. You are building movement into a normally sedentary life.

Is your sleep disturbed? Are you worrying at night? Try doing deep relaxation before bed or if you awaken in the middle of the night. Consciously let go before you sleep.

Use imagery to let go of worry. Imagine that the meeting will go well and you got that promotion or sale, that your life is easeful and your mind is peaceful. When you are having trouble falling asleep try counting your many blessings. Have peaceful dreams or a dreamless sleep.

Hopefully these solutions will enable you to incorporate Yoga practices in your life, making it more efficient and enjoyable. The regular and formal Yoga practice is very important. It is the roots of the tree. Make them strong and deep.

You be the master chef. I have presented all the ingredients; now it is your turn to mix them together into a delicious tasty lifestyle that is unique to you alone.

As you mold your future by inspiring yourself to health and well-being, infuse your life with a sense of peace and dynamic stillness to handle each new challenge with ease and integrity. More energy will then be available for that which is important to you and gives you joy.

You will then be able to honor the center of your being as truth, light, and love beyond everyday thoughts and feelings. In those moments when you embrace that place in yourself, you are able to honor it in others. You will then radiate that joy to everyone you meet.

INDEX

ABOUT THE AUTHOR

NISCHALA JOY DEVI is internationally renowned and has been teaching all aspects of Yoga and meditation for over twenty-five years. She has a way of presenting the timeless teachings of Yoga that is down to earth and practical at the same time as it is uplifting and inspiring. Her dynamic delivery and deep inner conviction empower each individual.

Nischala is invited all over the world to conduct seminars, lectures, and workshops on Yoga and its use in healing and stress management. She spends some time each year teaching in Europe, helping students from many disciplines develop their own healing potential. She is a tutor for the German, Belgian, British, Italian, and European Yoga unions. She was invited to teach—and was the keynote speaker—at the First International Conference of Yoga in Moscow and the Uniting of the Americas through Yoga in Costa Rica.

Nischala helped develop and was the primary instructor for the Basic and Advanced Teachers Training Program of Integral Yoga International. She has trained teachers in the United States, Europe, Canada, Australia—more than eight hundred teachers worldwide.

Before coming to Yoga, she was educated and worked in traditional medicine for fifteen years. It was then she started to see a lack of spirit in the medical field. She felt there was a missing aspect and she wanted to find it. Her search led her through many spiritual paths until she found Yoga. During her eighteen years as a monk, she started to merge the ancient wisdom of Yoga with some modern medical technique. The great results she saw subsequently led her to work with people who had life-threatening diseases, in particular, cancer and heart disease.

In 1985, she cofounded the award-winning Commonweal Cancer Help Program in California.

Nischala Devi was one of the early collaborators in developing the Yoga portion for The Lifestyle Heart Trial, which later was the inspiration for Dr. Dean Ornish's Program for Reversing Heart Disease. Nischala Devi served as the director of stress management, training the stress management specialists (Yoga teachers) for The Multicenter Lifestyle Heart Trial, the hospital-based version of the Reversing Heart Disease program. For seven years, she also taught Yoga and lectured in the weeklong residential lifestyle retreats of the Ornish programs.

She serves as advisory board member for The International Association of Yoga Therapists and is an advisor and consultant lecturer for Satyam Vidya Centre for Integral Studies, Gloucestershire, England.

Nischala has been awarded grants from the Hale Fund and the Rockefeller Fund respectively for her continuing service in Yoga and life-threatening diseases.

She produced the Abundant Well-Being audiocassette series. *Relax, Move & Heal,* a movement and relaxation tape; *Deep Relaxation; Sojourn to Healing,* on imagery; and *Dynamic Stillness,* on meditation, are tapes that have been used in the Dr. Dean Ornish program, the Commonweal Cancer Help Program, and many other people wishing to heal or enhance their well-being. These tapes allow her healing and stress-relieving techniques to touch people all over the world.

Nischala's work with people suffering with life-threatening disease has led her to develop *Yoga of the Heart,* a training program for Yoga teachers to adapt the ancient teaching of Yoga for cardiac disease so many can be helped by these teachings.

Her realistic approach and unique openness to the problems of today and the combining of spirituality with the modern world allow her to relate easily to all types of people in many different circumstances all over the globe. This special gift gives her the freedom to expand beyond boundaries and limitations of any one tradition or technique, enabling her to touch people's hearts.

NISCHALA JOY DEVI
P.O. Box 346
Fairfax, CA 94978-0346
Tel/Fax: 415-459-5336
E-mail: nd@abundantwellbeing.com
abundantwellbeing.com